Practical Clinical Endodontics

Acknowledgements

Our thanks to Sheila Lumley for her assistance in preparation of the diagrams in this book.

Commissioning Editor: Michael Parkinson
Project Development Manager: Sarah Keer-Keer
Project Manager: Frances Affleck
Designer: Stewart Larking
Illustrator: Cactus Design and Illustration

Practical Clinical Endodontics

Philip Lumley BDS FDS RCPS MDentSc PhD FDSRCS FDSRCSEd

Professor of Endodontology, Honorary Consultant in Restorative Dentistry,
Birmingham Dental Hospital and School

Nick Adams BDS MSc MRDRCS(Eng)

Specialist in Endodontics,
Clinical Lecturer and Honorary Associate Specialist in Endodontics,
Birmingham Dental Hospital and School

Phillip Tomson BDS MFDS RCSEd MFDS RCSEng

Clinical Lecturer in Restorative Dentistry,
Birmingham Dental Hospital and School

Birmingham Dental Hospital and School,
St Chads Queensway,
Birmingham, UK

Series editor

F.J. Trevor Burke

Professor of Dental Primary Care
University of Birmingham School of Dentistry

CHURCHILL LIVINGSTONE

ELSEVIER

Edinburgh London New York Oxford Philadelphia St Louis Sydney Toronto 2006

CHURCHILL
LIVINGSTONE
ELSEVIER

First published 2006

ISBN 0443074828

British Library Cataloguing in Publication Data
A catalogue record for this book is available from the British Library

Library of Congress Cataloging in Publication Data
A catalog record for this book is available from the Library of Congress

Note
Knowledge and best practice in this field are constantly changing. As new research and experience broaden our knowledge, changes in practice, treatment and drug therapy may become necessary or appropriate. Readers are advised to check the most current information provided (i) on procedures featured or (ii) by the manufacturer of each product to be administered, to verify the recommended dose or formula, the method and duration of administration, and contraindications. It is the responsibility of the practitioner, relying on their own experience and knowledge of the patient, to make diagnoses, to determine dosages and the best treatment for each individual patient, and to take all appropriate safety precautions. To the fullest extent of the law, neither the publisher nor the authors assume any liability for any injury and/or damage to persons or property arising out of or related to any use of the material contained in this book.

The Publisher

Printed and bound by CPI Group (UK) Ltd, Croydon, CR0 4YY

Transferred to Digital Print 2011

The publisher's policy is to use **paper manufactured from sustainable forests**

Preface

The microbial aetiology of endodontic disease is well established and becoming increasingly well understood. The past decade has seen major changes in the equipment and techniques available for the management of pulpal and periradicular disease. However these developments, although helpful, have arguably resulted in the emphasis of management of endodontic disease moving from a biological to a mechanical basis.

This book brings the biological concepts and new techniques together. Patients are becoming increasingly reluctant to lose teeth and this has led to the practitioner being faced increasingly with demands for endodontic therapy. The text provides an overview of the disease processes and explains many of the new technologies available for addressing these established biological problems.

The text is not intended to be comprehensively inclusive but is suitable for dental practitioners, junior hospital staff and undergraduate dental students. It is comprehensively illustrated with the authors' own cases and references towards further reading are presented at the end of each chapter. Clinical aspects of endodontic disease are discussed, including aetiology, clinical features and management. Key aspects of primary treatment, root canal re-treatment and periradicuar surgery are presented.

PJL
NA
PLT

Contents

1 The scientific basis for treating endodontic infection

THE IDENTIFICATION OF BACTERIA INVOLVED IN ENDODONTIC INFECTION

Microorganisms (Fig. 1.1) have long been implicated in the pathogenesis of pulpal and periradicular disease. In 1894, Miller[1] described bacteria in pulp chambers and root canals and also reported that intraradicular bacteria were different from those in the pulp chamber. It was not until 1966, however, that bacteria were conclusively shown to cause pulpal necrosis and periradicular inflammation when Kakehashi et al[2] exposed pulps in both gnotobiotic and conventional rats for 42 days. Pulpal healing occurred in the gnotobiotes compared to necrosis and abscess formation in the conventional animals (Fig. 1.2). In 1966, Moller[3] described a technique which allowed samples of bacteria to be maintained and subsequently cultured in the laboratory. The advent of this technique led to subsequent identification of anaerobic bacteria involved in endodontic infection.

Bacterial penetration

Pulp

It has been shown that insignificant pulpal changes occur when bacteria have penetrated to within 1.1 mm of the pulp; however, irreversible damage occurred if they penetrated to within 0.5 mm.[4] Further clinical studies involving traumatized non-vital teeth with intact pulp chambers showed that periradicular inflammation only developed in teeth from which bacteria could be isolated.[5,6] Trowbridge and Stevens[7] demonstrated that bacteria can enter the pulp and have proposed that this may be via:

- a deep carious lesion
- exposure of dentinal tubules or pulp during restorative procedures
- exposure of the pulp as a result of tooth fracture
- exposure of accessory canals by deep periodontal pockets.

Additional routes of entry include blood communication via the gingivae and periodontal ligament or anachoresis.

Dentine

Bacteria (predominantly anaerobic) have been shown to have the potential to invade root canal dentine in teeth with necrotic pulps. Invasion of predentine was found to be common but hard tissue invasion rarer. A number of studies have used light and electron microscopy to investigate the distribution of bacteria in the root canal. Nair[8] and Nair et al[9] demonstrated bacteria densely filling Howship's lacunae on the root canal wall and also suspended in the canal lumen if it was filled with fluid. Rod-shaped bacteria dominated the root canal flora, but cocci, filaments and spirochaetes were also seen, including 'corncob'-like structures formed by cocci and filaments, and deposits resembling bacterial plaque. Bacterial penetration of the dentinal tubules could vary between 10 and 150 μm.

TYPES OF BACTERIA

More than 300 bacterial groups or species of bacteria are recognized as normal inhabitants of the oral cavity and all theoretically have the capacity to invade the root canal space during and after pulp necrosis. The microflora of infected root canals, however, include a restricted group of species when compared to the total oral flora and most have the capacity to initiate periradicular inflammation. Pulps of monkey teeth were infected with indigenous oral bacteria from saliva, which sealed the cavities after 7 days for varying periods of time from 3 months to 3 years. Samples were taken from the apical region of the tooth at the end of each period. After 6 months, obligate anaerobes outnumbered facultative anaerobes and, as the time period increased, the proportion of obligate anaerobes increased further.

Combinations of bacterial strains originally isolated from an endogenously infected root canal inoculated

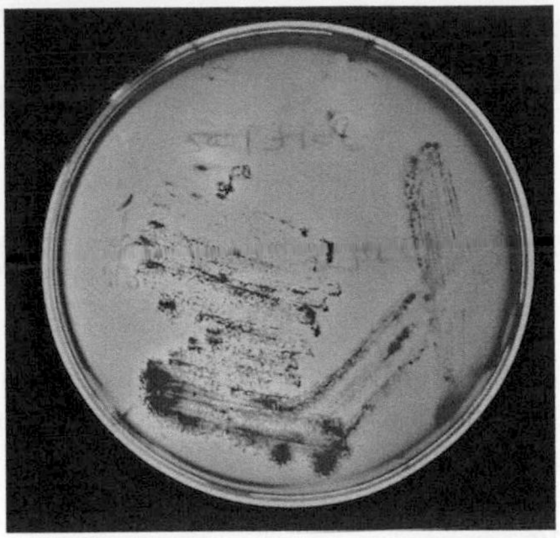

Figure 1.1 Bacteria isolated from root canal infection.

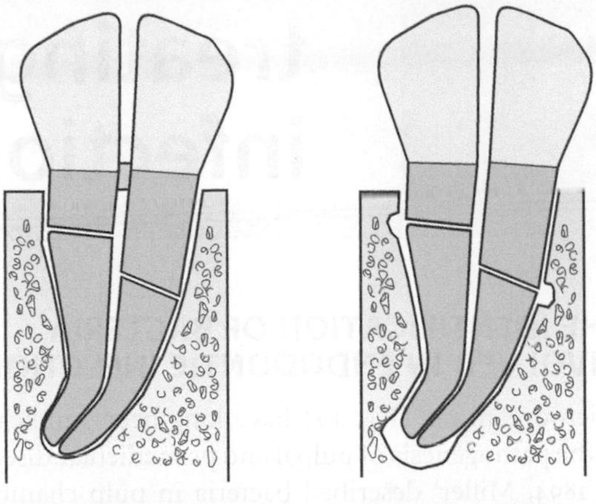

Figure 1.2 Diagrammatic representation of Kakehashi's experiment.

Table 1.1 Common pathogens isolated from the root canals

	Gram-positive cocci	Gram-positive rods	Gram-negative cocci	Gram-negative rods	Others
Facultative anaerobes	Streptococcus Enterococcus	Actinomyces Lactobacillus	Neisseria	Capnocytophaga Eikenella	Candida
Obligate anaerobes	Streptococcus Peptostreptococcus	Actinomyces Lactobacillus Eubacterium	Veillonella	Porphyromonas Prevotella Fusobacterium Campylobacter	

into canals with devitalized tissue resulted in a flora dominated by anaerobic bacteria. When these bacteria were inoculated in monoculture the majority were not recovered after 6 months, the exception being enterococci. On average, 8–15 species were isolated per tooth. This demonstrates that root canal infection is dynamic, with selective mechanisms operating in favour of the growth and survival of specific microorganisms. The existence of many microorganisms in the root canal would imply certain interactions between the bacterial population which affect their growth and physiological behaviour.

The advent of molecular techniques to examine the root canal flora has led to the discovery of previously uncultured microorganisms. A study comparing the bacterial isolate from a root canal using both culturing and molecular techniques identified a total of 44 species, 23 by culturing and 23 by polymerase chain reaction (PCR) cloning, with five species being common to both techniques.[10] Table 1.1 shows the common microorganisms isolated from the root canal.

HOST DEFENCE REACTION

Bacteria and their by-products elicit a host defence reaction which initially consists of a non-specific response. This may result in vasodilation, formation of tissue fluid and cellular exudate, i.e. polymorphonuclear leucocytes and macrophages, and activation of the kinin and complement systems with release of histamine, plasmins, Hageman factor, prostaglandins and leukotrienes. The specific host response consists of cellular and humoral immunity and involves T and B lymphocytes, lymphokines, plasma cells and immunoglobulins.

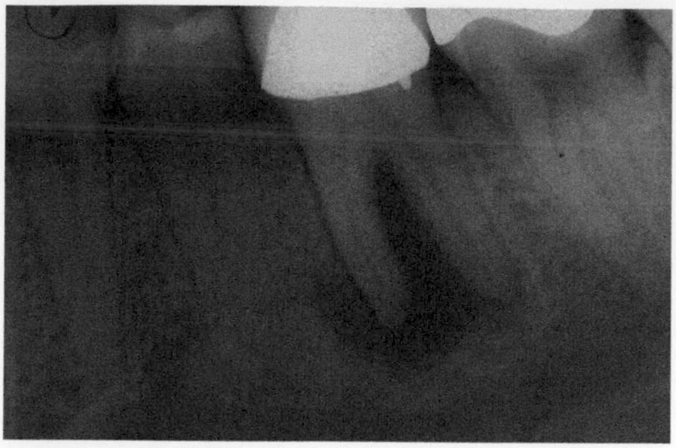

Figure 1.3 Preoperative radiograph of LL6 with evidence of periapical pathology.

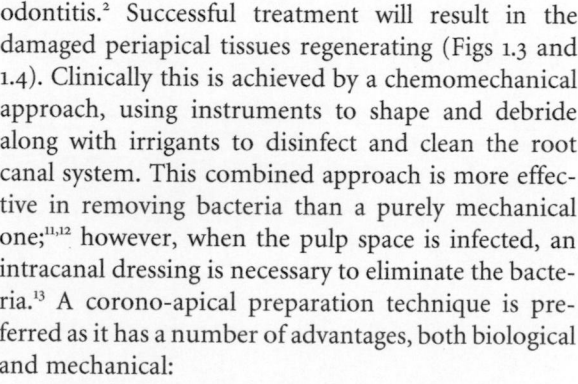

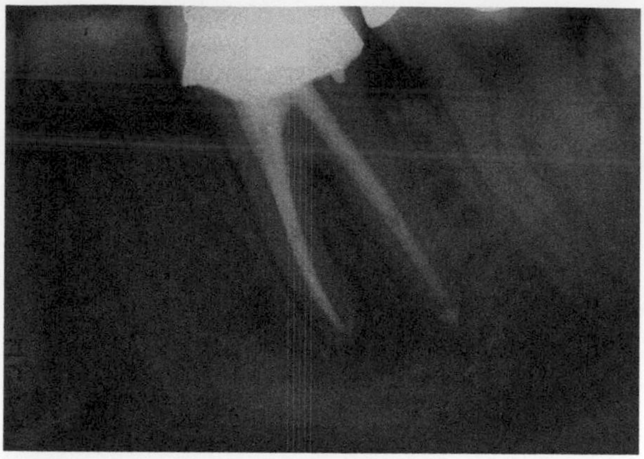

Figure 1.4 The tooth illustrated in Figure 1.3 at 5-month follow-up; note reduction in the radiolucent area in the periapical tissues.

Microorganism resistance

Microorganisms are capable of resisting the host defences by a number of mechanisms. Certain non-encapsulated species can produce a capsule in vivo which will enable the organisms to resist phagocytosis and intracellular killing. They can also produce soluble short chain fatty acids which inhibit polymorphonucleocyte functions such as chemotaxis, degranulation and phagocytosis. Enzymes that hydrolyse immunoglobulins, complement and tissue proteins such as collagen may also be produced. Lipopolysaccharide (LPS) is a component of the outermost membrane of the cell wall of Gram-negative anaerobic bacteria, which are commonly found in root canal infections. LPS concentration is significantly higher on the pulpal compared to the cementum surface of the root and there is a strong correlation between LPS levels and the presence of exudation and radiolucent areas.

TREATMENT

From the clinical perspective the aim of endodontic treatment is to remove bacteria from the root canal system as it has been shown that they are the cause of pulpal inflammation, necrosis and periapical periodontitis.[2] Successful treatment will result in the damaged periapical tissues regenerating (Figs 1.3 and 1.4). Clinically this is achieved by a chemomechanical approach, using instruments to shape and debride along with irrigants to disinfect and clean the root canal system. This combined approach is more effective in removing bacteria than a purely mechanical one;[11,12] however, when the pulp space is infected, an intracanal dressing is necessary to eliminate the bacteria.[13] A corono-apical preparation technique is preferred as it has a number of advantages, both biological and mechanical:

- biologically, the majority of bacteria are removed from the root canal system prior to apical instrumentation
- mechanically there is less stress applied to the instruments during apical preparation which can make tactile determination of the apical constriction easier.[14]

These important aspects should be considered alongside the use of appropriate antibacterial irrigation regimes and intervisit dressings to give the optimum outcome of clinical treatment.

REFERENCES

1. Miller WD. An introduction to the study of the bacteriology of the dental pulp. Dental Cosmos 1894; 36: 505–528.
2. Kakehashi S, Stanley HR, Fitzgerald RJ. The effects of surgical exposures of dental pulps in germ-free and conventional laboratory rats. Oral Surg Oral Pathol 1966; 20: 340–349.
3. Moller AJR. Microbial examination of root canals and periapical tissues in human teeth. Methodological studies. Odont Tidskr 1966; 74(Suppl): 1–380.
4. Reeves S, Stanley HR. The relationship of bacterial penetration and pulpal pathosis in carious teeth. Oral Pathol 1965; 22: 59–65.

5. Sundqvist G. Bacteriologic studies of necrotic dental pulps. PhD Thesis, Umea University 1976; Odontol Dissertation no 7: 1–94.
6. Bergenholtz G. Microorganisms from necrotic pulps of traumatized teeth. Odont Revy 1974; 25: 347–358.
7. Trowbridge HO, Stevens BH. Microbiologic and pathologic aspects of pulpal and periapical disease. Curr Opin Dent 1992; 2: 85–92.
8. Nair PNR. Light and electron microscopic studies of root canal flora and periapical lesions. J Endod 1987; 13: 29–39.
9. Nair PNR, Sjogren U, Krey G, Kahnberg KE, Sundqvist G. Intraradicular bacteria and fungi in root filled, asymptomatic human teeth with periapical lesions: a long term light and electron microscope follow-up study. J Endod 1990; 16: 580–588.
10. Gulabivala K. Personal communication.
11. Bystrom A, Sundqvist G. Bacteriologic evaluation of the efficacy of mechanical root canals instrumentation in endodontic therapy. Scand J Dent Res 1981; 89: 321–328.
12. Bystrom A, Sundqvist G. Bacteriologic evaluation of the effect of 0.5 percent sodium hypochlorite in endodontic therapy. Oral Surg Oral Med Oral Pathol 1983; 55: 307–312.
13. Bystrom A, Claesson R, Sundqvist G. The antibacterial effect of camphorated paramonochlorophenol, camphorated phenol and calcium hydroxide in the treatment of infected root canals. Endod Dent Traumatol 1985; 1: 170–175.
14. Stabholz A, Rotstein I, Torabinejad M. Effect of preflaring on tactile detection of the apical constriction. J Endod 1995; 21: 92–94.

2 Disease processes

Pulpal or periradicular inflammation results from irritation or injury, usually from bacterial, mechanical or chemical sources.

- *Bacteria* — usually from dental caries — are the main sources of injury to the pulpal and periradicular tissues and enter either directly or through dentine tubules. The link between bacteria and pulpal and periradicular disease is well established: in the absence of bacteria, periradicular pathology does not develop. Modes of entry for bacteria other than caries are summarized in Box 2.1.
- *Mechanical irritants* — examples of mechanical irritation include excessive orthodontic forces and over-instrumentation by root canal instruments.
- *Chemical irritants* — periradicular irritation may occur from irrigating solutions, phenolic-based intracanal medicaments or extrusion of root canal filling materials.

PULP DISEASE

Irritation from bacterial, mechanical or chemical sources causes some degree of inflammation. The response of the pulp depends on the severity of the insult and may result in either a reversible inflammatory response or an irreversible one that will eventually proceed to pulp necrosis.

CLASSIFICATION OF PULP DISEASE

There is an inconsistent correlation between clinical symptoms and histological findings in pulpal disease.[1] Diagnoses are therefore usually based on patient symptoms and clinical findings.[2] Pulpal disease may result in changes to both the soft and hard tissues.

Soft tissue changes

Reversible pulpitis

This is a transient condition which may be precipitated by caries, erosion, attrition, abrasion, operative procedures, scaling or mild trauma. The symptoms of reversible pulpitis are summarized in Box 2.2. Treatment involves covering exposed dentine, removing the stimulus or dressing the tooth as appropriate. Reversible pulpitis may progress to an irreversible situation.

Irreversible pulpitis

Irreversible pulpitis usually occurs as a result of more severe insults of the type listed above and, typically, it may develop as a progression from a reversible state. The symptoms of irreversible pulpitis are summarized in Box 2.3. Treatment involves either root canal therapy or extraction of the tooth.

Hyperplastic pulpitis

This form of irreversible pulpitis is also known as a pulp polyp. It occurs as a result of proliferation of chronically inflamed young pulp tissue. Treatment involves root canal therapy or extraction.

Pulp necrosis

Pulp necrosis occurs as the end result of irreversible pulpitis. Treatment involves root canal therapy or extraction.

Hard tissue changes

Pulp calcification

Physiological secondary dentine is formed continuously after tooth eruption and the completion of root development. It is deposited on the floor and ceiling of the pulp chamber rather than the walls and with time can result in occlusion of the pulp chamber. Tertiary dentine is laid down in response to environmental stimuli as reactionary or reparative dentine.

Box 2.1 Modes of entry of bacteria into the pulp other than caries

- Exposure of the tubules or pulp during restorative procedures
- Periodontal disease (dentine tubules, furcal canals, lateral canals)
- Tooth substance loss such as erosion, attrition and abrasion
- Trauma with or without pulpal exposure
- Developmental anomalies
- Anachoresis (the passage of microorganisms into the root canal system from the blood stream)

Box 2.2 Symptoms of reversible pulpitis

- Pain does not linger after the stimulus is removed
- Pain is difficult to localize (the pulp contains only nociceptive and not proprioceptive fibres)
- Normal periradicular radiographic appearance
- Teeth are not tender to percussion (unless occlusal trauma is present)

Box 2.3 Symptoms of irreversible pulpitis

- Pain may develop spontaneously or from stimuli
- In the latter stages heat may be more significant
- Response lasts from minutes to hours
- When the periodontal ligament becomes involved, the pain will be localized
- A widened periodontal ligament may be seen radiographically in the later stages (see Fig. 2.1)

Reactionary dentine is a response to a mild noxious stimulus whereas reparative dentine is deposited directly beneath the path of injured dentinal tubules as a response to strong noxious stimuli. Treatment is dependent upon the pulpal symptoms.

Internal resorption

Occasionally, pulpal inflammation may cause changes that result in dentinoclastic activity. Such changes result in resorption of dentine and clinically a pink spot (Fig. 2.2A) may be seen in the later stages if the lesion is coronal. Radiographic examination (Fig. 2.2B) reveals a punched-out outline that is seen to be continuous with the rest of the pulp cavity. Root canal therapy will result in arrest of the resorptive process; however, if destruction is very advanced, extraction may be required.

It should be borne in mind that pulpal inflammation is not static and does not progress in an orderly manner from one state to another; simultaneous chronic and acute inflammation is possible.[3]

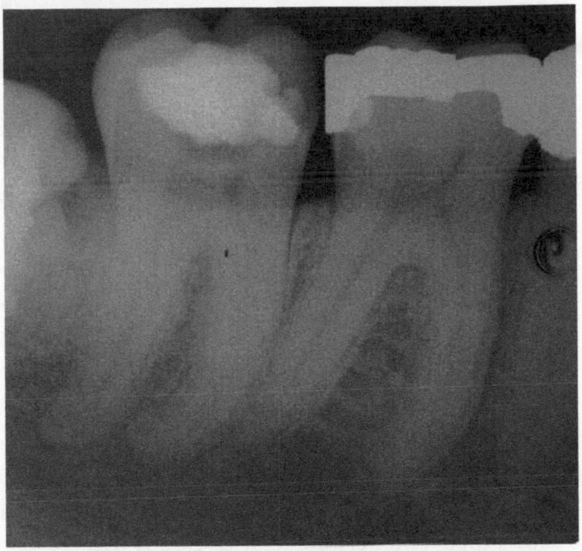

Figure 2.1 A widened periodontal ligament space.

CLASSIFICATION OF PERIAPICAL DISEASE

Acute apical periodontitis

Causes of acute apical periodontitis include occlusal trauma, egress of bacteria from infected pulp, toxins from necrotic pulp, chemicals, irrigants or over-instrumentation in root canal therapy. Clinically, the tooth is tender to biting and widening of the periodontal space may be seen on a radiograph. Treatment depends on the pulpal diagnosis, and thus may range from occlusal adjustment to root canal therapy or extraction.

Chronic apical periodontitis

Chronic apical periodontitis occurs as a result of pulp necrosis. Affected teeth do not respond to pulp sensi-

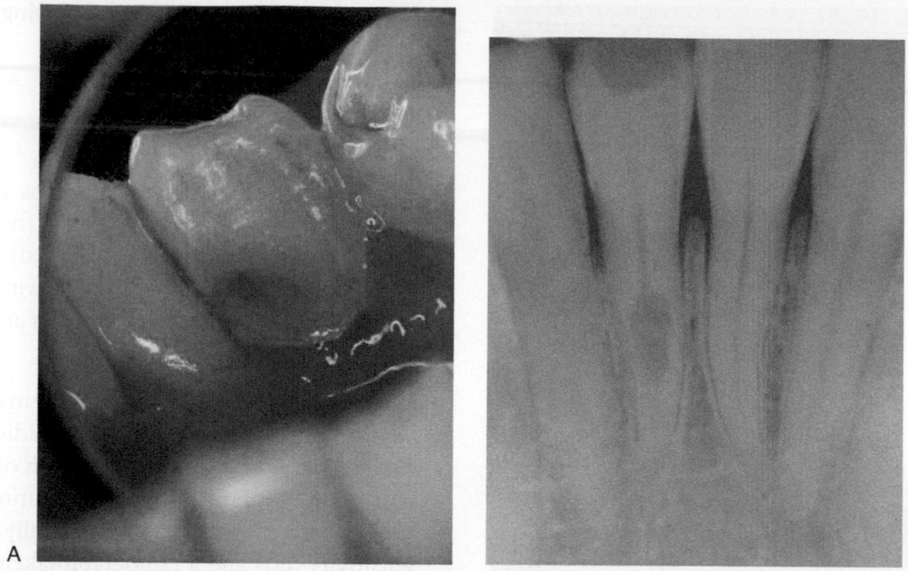

Figure 2.2 Clinical photograph (A) and radiograph (B) of two different teeth with internal resorption.

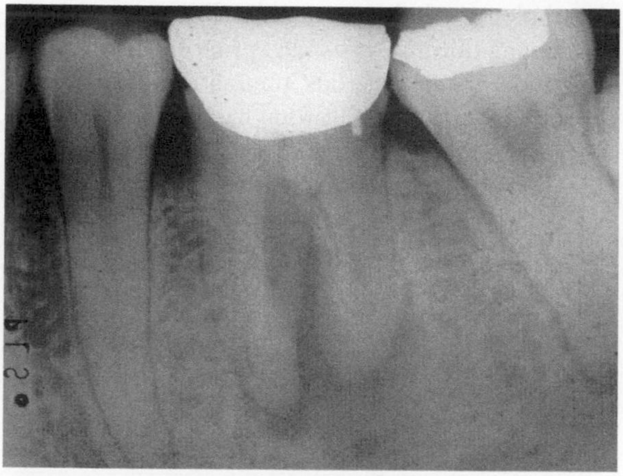

Figure 2.3 A tooth with apical periodontitis.

tivity tests. Tenderness to biting, if present, is usually mild; however, some tenderness may be noted to palpation over the root apex. Radiographic appearance is varied, ranging from minimal widening of the periodontal ligament space to a large area of destruction of periapical tissues (Fig. 2.3). Treatment involves root canal therapy or extraction.

Condensing osteitis

Condensing osteitis is a variant of chronic apical periodontitis and represents a diffuse increase in trabecular bone in response to irritation. Radiographically, a concentric radiopaque area is seen around the offending root. Treatment is required only if symptoms/pulpal diagnosis indicate a need.

Acute apical abscess

An acute apical abscess is a severe inflammatory response to microorganisms or their irritants that have leached out into the periradicular tissues. Symptoms vary from moderate discomfort or swelling to systemic involvement, such as raised temperature and malaise. Teeth involved are usually tender to both palpation and percussion. Radiographic changes are variable depending on the amount of periradicular destruction already present; however, there is usually a well-defined radiolucent area, as in many situations an acute apical abscess is an acute exacerbation of a chronic situation. One well-recognized event is that of a phoenix abscess — an acute exacerbation of a chronic situation during treatment.

Initial treatment of an acute apical abscess involves removal of the cause as soon as possible. Drainage should be established either by opening the tooth or by incision into a dependent swelling. An antibiotic or analgesics may need to be prescribed depending on the patient's condition. Once the acute symptoms have

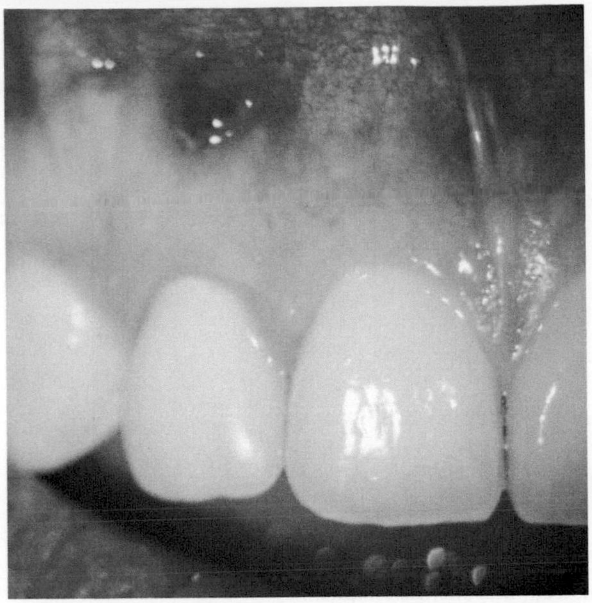

Figure 2.4 Intraoral sinus.

subsided then root canal therapy or extraction may be performed.

Chronic apical abscess

In such cases the abscess has formed a communication through which it discharges. The communication may be through a sinus intraorally (Fig. 2.4) or, less commonly, extraorally. Alternatively, the discharge may be along the periodontal ligament, and such cases mimic a periodontal pocket. Usually these communications or tracts heal spontaneously following root canal therapy or extraction.

RADIOGRAPHIC LESIONS OF NON-ENDODONTIC ORIGIN

Although lesions noted on radiographs are usually of endodontic origin this is not always the case. Other causes include normal anatomical structures, and benign or malignant lesions. The following lists are not exhaustive and readers should refer to an appropriate text on oral pathology:

- *Anatomical structures* — certain normal anatomical structures may mimic radiolucencies, e.g. maxillary sinus, mental foramen or nasopalatine foramen. In these situations the associated teeth will respond normally to pulp sensitivity tests and a radiograph taken from a different angle will reveal that the lesion is not so closely related to the root.
- *Benign lesions* that may mimic endodontic pathology include cementoma, fibrous dysplasia, ossifying fibroma, cysts (e.g. primordial, lateral periodontal, dentigerous, traumatic bone), central giant cell granuloma, central haemangioma and ameloblastoma. Usually in such situations the lamina dura will be intact around the teeth and final diagnosis relies on appropriate biopsy.
- *Malignant lesions* to be aware of include squamous cell carcinoma, osteosarcoma, chondrosarcoma and multiple myeloma. These lesions are usually associated with rapid hard tissue destruction.

REFERENCES

1. Dummer PMH, Hicks R, Hows D. Clinical signs and symptoms in pulp disease. Int Endod J 1980; 13: 27–35.
2. Montgomery S, Fergusson CD. Diagnosis, treatment planning and prognostic considerations. Dent Clin North Am 1986; 30: 533–548.
3. Seltzer S, Bender I, Zionitz M. The diagnosis of pulp inflammation: correlations between diagnostic data and actual histologic findings in the pulp. Oral Surg Oral Med Oral Pathol 1963; 66: 969–977.

3 History, diagnosis, case selection and treatment planning

The most common cause of orofacial pain is pulpal or periradicular disease. However, it should be remembered that the periodontium, sinuses, temporomandibular joints (TMJs), muscles of mastication, ears, nose, eyes, nerve and blood vessels may also be affected by lesions which can mimic pain of pulpal origin.

Successful endodontic diagnosis requires a systematic approach to the history and clinical examination, followed by the use of appropriate diagnostic aids.

HISTORY

Presenting complaint

The aim of this stage is to record the patient's symptoms or problems, preferably in their own words.

Medical history

An up-to-date medical history should be taken for each new patient or be updated for previously registered patients, dated and signed.

Dental history

The purpose of this stage is to gain a summary of current and past dental treatment. Such information may provide clues as to the source of the patient's complaints. It is also an opportunity to establish the patient's attitude towards dental health and treatment, as these findings may affect treatment decisions or planning.

Pain history

Initially, information is obtained by asking questions regarding the current problem(s). This examination is subjective; a list of frequently asked questions follows:

Location Occasionally a patient may identify the location of the pain; however, one must be cautious as pulpal pain may be referred to a different area. Pain may be felt in any of the orofacial structures.

Type and intensity of pain The patient may describe pain in many ways. Examples include sharp, dull, throbbing, stabbing, burning, electric shock-like, deep or superficial. The more the pain disrupts the patient's lifestyle because of its intensity, the more likely it is to be irreversible in origin.

Duration For how long after removal of the stimulus does the pain continue? The longer the pain continues after the stimulus, the more likely it is to be irreversible.

Stimulus Many different stimuli may initiate the pain; for example, hot, cold, sweet, biting and posture. Alternatively, the pain may be spontaneous. Special tests may be selected on the basis of what causes the main complaint.

Relief Pain-relieving factors, especially type and frequency of analgesics, antibiotics, and in some cases sipping cold drinks.

Provisional diagnosis

The history and identification of signs and symptoms may help the clinician to reach a provisional diagnosis. The clinical examination gathers the information necessary to confirm or modify this diagnosis.

CLINICAL EXAMINATION

Extraoral The patient's general appearance and well-being are assessed. A note is made of any swelling, redness or presence of extraoral sinuses (Figs 3.1 and 3.2). Lymph nodes are palpated for enlargement and/or tenderness. Muscles of mastication and TMJs are also palpated for tenderness and a note made of the degree of mouth opening.

Intraoral soft tissues All of the oral mucosa and gingival tissues are examined for discolouration, inflammatory change and pathology.

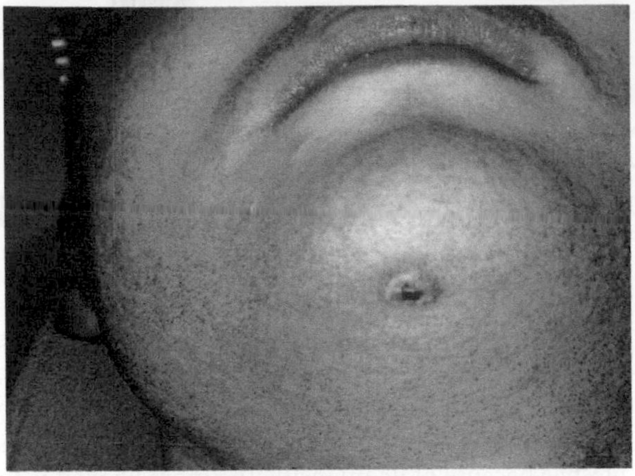

Figure 3.1 Extraoral sinus originating from necrotic lower incisors.

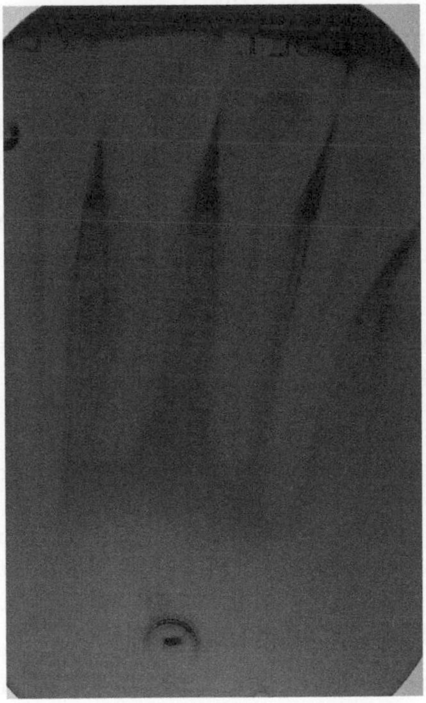

Figure 3.2 Radiograph of the lower incisors of the patient shown in Figure 3.1.

Periodontium A basic periodontal examination (BPE) is performed. An area for which a code 4 is recorded requires further periodontal assessment.

Intraoral (hard tissues) Teeth are examined for caries, large restorations, crowns, discolouration, fracture, attrition, abrasion, erosion and restorability.

Tooth-specific examination

Soft tissues

Redness The tissues surrounding the tooth are examined for redness.

Sinus tract exploration Where present, a sinus tract is noted and indicates the presence of a suppurative lesion (Fig. 3.3A). It may be possible to insert a gutta-percha point into the sinus and expose a radiograph to see which root the tract/point leads to (Fig. 3.3B).

Swelling The presence of swelling adjacent to the tooth is noted, and also whether it is hard or firm in nature.

Palpation This involves the palpation of the adjacent buccal and/or lingual mucosa. A positive response (tenderness) indicates that inflammation has spread within the cancellous bone and reached the cortical plate and underlying periosteum.

Percussion This refers to gently tapping or pressing the occlusal or lateral surface of a tooth. A painful response indicates periradicular inflammation.

Periodontium

Pockets If indicated from the BPE, a detailed pocket chart is undertaken. Detailed periodontal probing around suspect teeth may reveal a sulcus within normal limits. However, on occasion, deeper pocketing will be noted. A narrow defect may be an indication of a root fracture or an endodontic lesion draining through the gingival crevice (Fig. 3.4). Broader-based lesions are usually an indication of disease of periodontal origin. Pulp sensitivity testing may help to distinguish between an infection of endodontic or periodontal origin when an endodontic/periodontal communication is present.

Mobility A mirror handle is placed on the side of the tooth and a note made of the degree of movement. Up to 1 mm scores 1; over 1 mm, 2; vertically mobile teeth, 3.

Bleeding on probing This is noted and related to other periodontal findings. Any discharge of pus is also recorded.

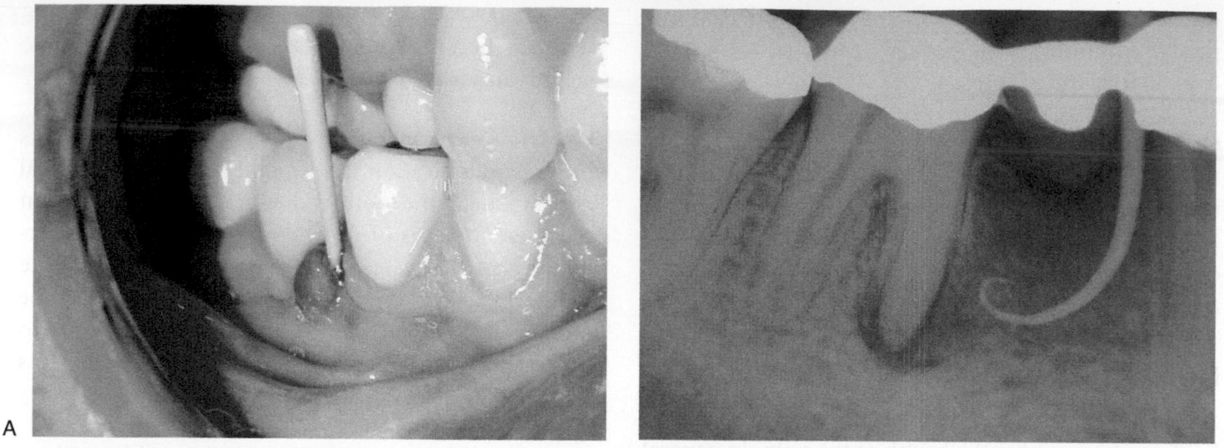

Figure 3.3 (A) Intraoral sinus with gutta-percha point tracing sinus tract; (B) Radiograph of previous.

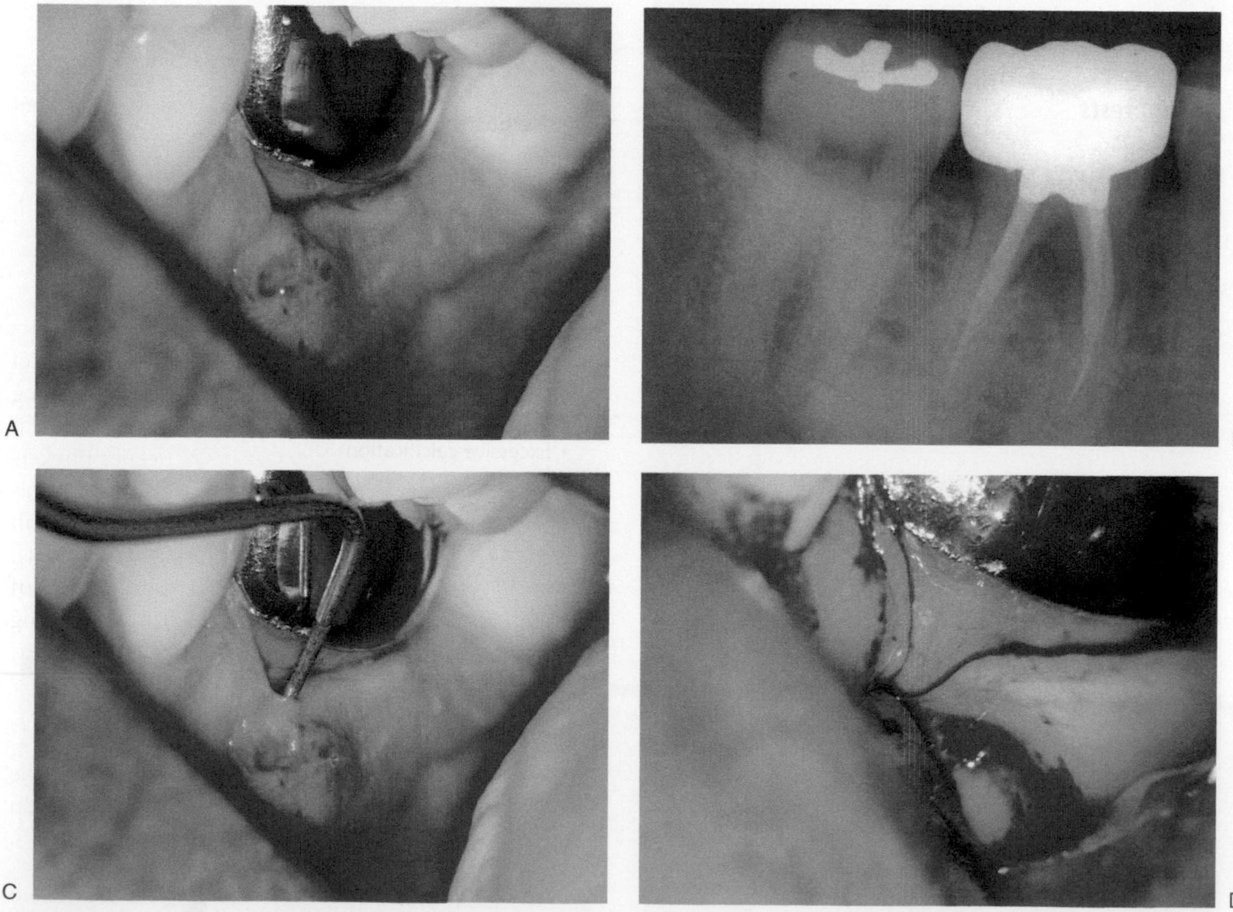

Figure 3.4 (A) Discharge opposite lower first molar; (B) radiograph of tooth; (C) a deep isolated pocket indicating the possibility of a root fracture; (D) gingiva reflected showing root fracture.

Recession Recession may also be noted and, if appropriate, combined with pocket depths to record the overall attachment loss.

Occlusal analysis It is important to examine suspect teeth for interferences on the retruded arc of closure, intercuspal position and lateral excursions. Interferences in any of these positions could result in a degree of occlusal trauma and institute acute apical periodontitis.

Diagnostic tests

All such tests have their limitations and can be unreliable in determining the health of the pulp. In general the tests used are more accurate in determining that a tooth is healthy, rather than has pathology associated with it.[1] Therefore, they require care in the way they are performed and interpreted. The objective is to find the tooth that is causing the discomfort. In general, healthy or control, teeth are tested first.

Special tests

Pulp sensitivity tests These determine the response to stimuli and may identify the offending tooth. It is usual to try to mimic the stimuli that initiate the pain.

Thermal tests

- *Cold test* — Endo Ice (Fig. 3.5) spray on a cotton pledget, ice or dry ice sticks may be used to mimic cold stimuli.

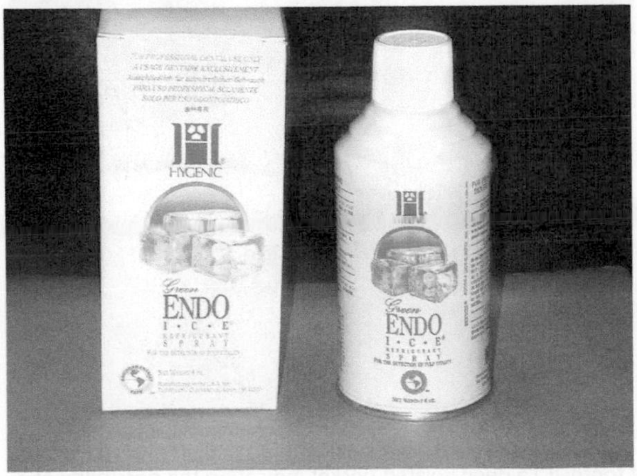

Figure 3.5 Endo Ice.

- *Hot test* — hot gutta-percha or hot water after the application of a rubber dam may be used to mimic hot stimuli.

Electric pulp test (Fig. 3.6) These instruments provide an indication as to whether or not there is vital nerve tissue in the tooth; it does not give an indication of different stages of degeneration, or provide information on the state of the blood flow through the tooth. In other words, no diagnostic data can be obtained other than a positive or negative response to the test.[2] It is also important to realize that false results can occur (see Box 3.1).

Transillumination Transillumination with a fibre-optic light can be useful in the diagnosis of cracks in teeth (Fig. 3.7).

Box 3.1 Causes of false vitality test results

False positive

- Contact with metallic restoration leading to contact with adjacent tooth or gingival sulcus
- Failure to isolate the tooth properly
- Anxiety
- Liquefaction necrosis leading to conduction at periodontal ligament

False negative

- Patient premedicated
- Inadequate contact
- Trauma
- Excessive calcification
- Immature apex
- Partial necrosis

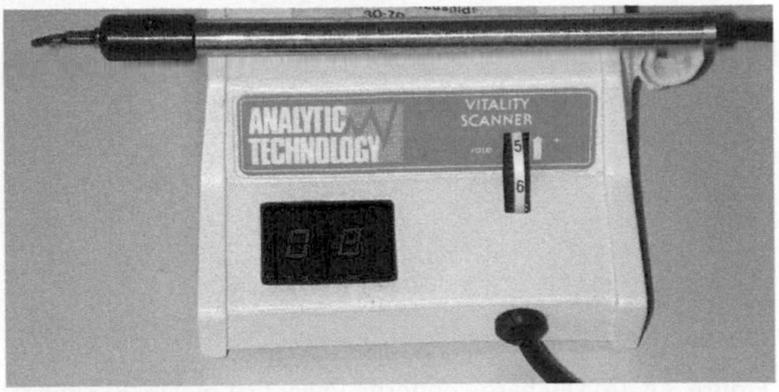

Figure 3.6 Electric pulp tester (Analytic Technology).

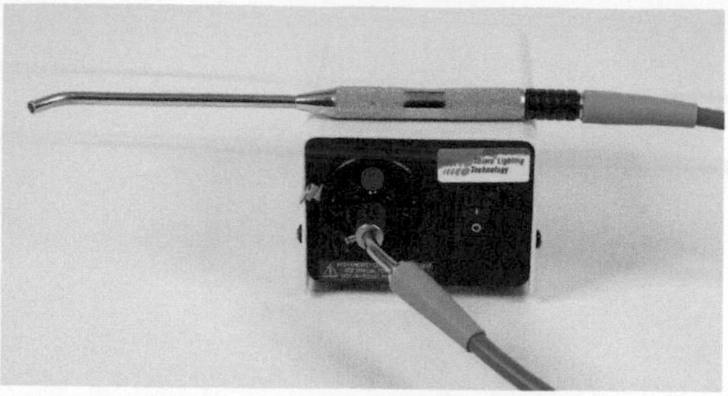

Figure 3.7 Fibreoptic transilluminator.

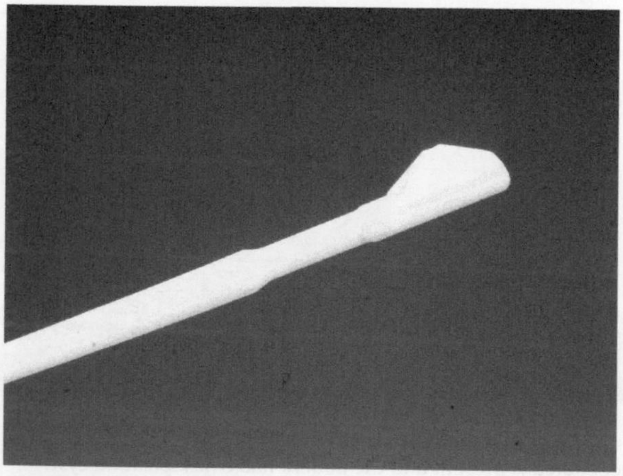

Figure 3.8 Tooth slooth.

Fracture detection Cracks may not be visible initially and the use of a piece of rubber dam (to bite on) between the teeth may aid diagnosis. A plastic bite stick ('tooth slooth' or 'frac finder', Fig. 3.8) is introduced to allow each cusp tip to be checked in turn; typically, the pain occurs on release of biting pressure.

Selective anaesthesia This can be useful in cases of referred pain, helping to distinguish whether the source of pain is mandibular or maxillary in origin. It is less useful for distinguishing pain from adjacent teeth as the anaesthetic solution may diffuse laterally.

Test cavity Occasionally, as a last resort, an access cavity may be cut into dentine without local anaesthesia as an additional way of sensitivity testing. However, it is unclear what additional diagnostic information can be gained from this procedure.

Radiographs Radiographs should be taken using film holders (Fig. 3.9) with a paralleling technique and viewed using an appropriate viewer, with magnification as necessary. They will not show early signs of pulpitis as there is no periodontal widening at this stage of pulpal degeneration. Radiographs may provide much important information to help confirm a diagnosis but should not be used alone. Radiographic findings may include the loss of lamina dura (laterally or apically) or a frank periradicular radiolucency (Fig. 3.10). Alternatively, radiographs may show pulp chamber or root canal calcification, which may explain reduced responses to pulp sensitivity testing, thus emphasizing the need for considering using more than one test. More rarely, radiographic examination may reveal tooth/root resorptive defects. A checklist for radiographic assessment is presented in Box 3.2.

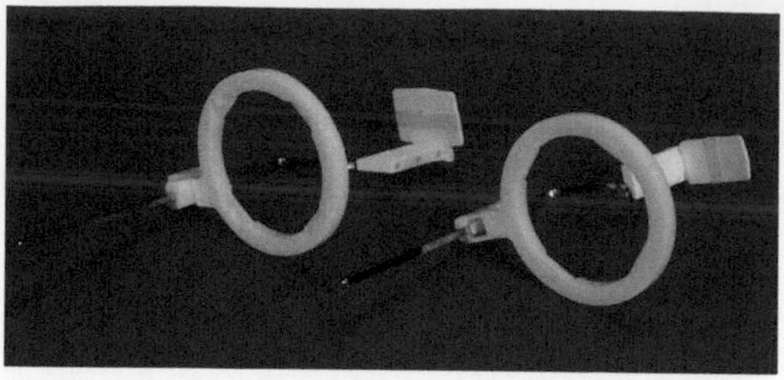

Figure 3.9 Film holders for use with paralleling technique.

Box 3.2 Checklist for radiographic assessment

- Periodontal bone support
- Caries
- Crown shape and size
- Proximity of restorations to pulp chamber
- Quality of restorations including coronal seal
- The size of the pulp chamber ± calcifications
- Crown : root ratio
- The number of roots
- Root anatomy
- Canal anatomy
- Canal calcification
- Root end proximity to important structures
- Presence of lesions of endodontic origin periradicularly or furcally
- Root fractures
- Extra root canals
- Resorptive defects
- Quality and effectiveness of previous treatment
- Root filling materials used
- Presence of pins/posts
- Iatrogenic complications

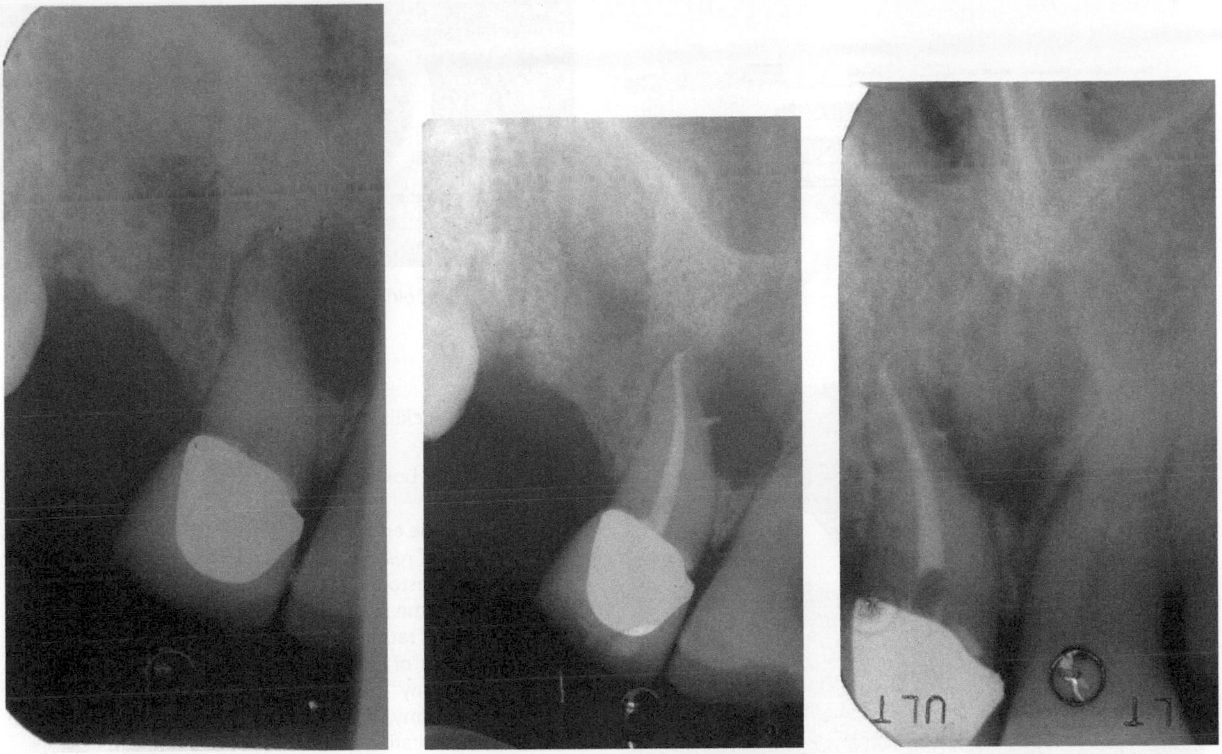

A B C

Figure 3.10 (A) Preoperative radiograph of tooth 21. A large radiolucent area is present and the patient had a nasopalatine cyst removed 12 months previously. (B) Radiograph following the completion of root canal therapy on 21. Note the presence of a lateral canal. (C) 12 month follow-up radiograph showing a reduction in the size of the radiolucent area following root canal therapy on 21.

DIAGNOSIS

Following this systematic approach to history taking and the application of appropriate special tests, it will usually be possible to make a diagnosis of the pulpal and periradicular problems. Such diagnoses have been covered previously and include reversible pulpitis, irreversible pulpitis, pulp necrosis, resorptive changes, acute and chronic apical periodontitis, and acute and chronic apical abscesses.

Because the correlation between clinical pulpal signs and symptoms and pulpal histology is poor, it is advisable to have two positive tests indicating pulpal pathology before embarking upon endodontic procedures or extraction. It is emphasized that it is important to record in the notes a pulpal and periradicular diagnosis upon which the treatment plan can be formulated. Despite this systematic and careful approach to diagnosis, there are occasions when arriving at an accurate diagnosis can be difficult.

Even after obtaining a thorough history and performing appropriate special tests, the clinician may still be unsure as to whether the pain is of dental origin. Endodontic treatment should not be performed on an ad hoc or 'hit and miss' basis. In cases of difficult diagnosis, a referral to an orofacial pain clinic, a neurosurgeon or an ENT specialist may be considered. A summary of examination and diagnostic procedures is presented in Box 3.3.

CASE SELECTION

Once a diagnosis has been reached, a plan needs to be formulated as to how to deal with the problem. The fact that an endodontic procedure is feasible is not sufficient justification for performing it. Endodontic treatment must be considered as part of an overall treatment plan in such a way that it represents the patient's best interests and wishes. The past dental history will have provided much information as to the

Box 3.3 Summary of examination and diagnostic procedures

What you can see
- Tooth restorable
- Tooth functional
- Redness present?
- Sinus present?
- Swelling present?

What you can test
- Sulcus tender to palpation
- Tooth tender to percussion
- Periodontal ligament
  — bleeding on probing (BOP)
  — mobility
  — pocket depth

Special tests
- Thermal
  — hot
  — cold
- Electric pulp test (EPT)
- Frac finder Tooth Slooth
- Transilluminate
- Radiographs
  — periapicals
  — bitewings
  — occlusal
  — orthopantomograph (OPT)

Diagnosis
- Pulp
  — vital
  — reversible pulpitis
  — irreversible pulpitis
  — necrotic
  — polyp
- Periradicular
  — normal
  — wide periodontal ligament
  — Radiolucent area, chronic apical periodontitis
  — Apical abcess, acute/chronic
  — condensing osteitis
  — ? root fracture

Treatment plan
- Monitor
- Orthograde root canal therapy
- Surgical root canal therapy
- Exploratory procedure
- Extract

patient's attitude towards treatment. Good endodontic treatment takes time, requiring a commitment from both clinician and patient.

TREATMENT PLANNING

Sequencing of treatment involves the management of pulpal or periodontal pain as a priority, and the extraction of unsavable teeth. Large carious lesions (Fig. 3.11) should be stabilized and a preventive regime, including periodontal therapy, instituted. Endodontic and restorative procedures can then be performed in a healthier environment and more predictable results obtained. A summary of some key aspects of endodontic diagnosis and case selection are presented in Box 3.4.

Indications for root canal therapy

Pulpal and periradicular disease

The most common indication for root canal therapy is pulpal or periradicular pathology. Elective root canal therapy may be performed for endodontic reasons. For example, teeth for which extensive restorative dentistry is planned and the subsequent tooth preparation would further stress a pulp of dubious prognosis. Alternatively, radiographs may show progressive calcification of the pulp space. This itself is not an indication for root canal therapy. However, such treatment may be performed if it is thought likely that the pulp space will be required for restorative purposes.

Restorative requirements

Occasionally, it may be decided to root treat a tooth electively for restorative reasons. Such situations include teeth which have fractured at the gingival level and for which post space is required for their restoration, and teeth that are going to be used as overdenture abutments.

Periodontal disease

If the periodontal lesion is of primary endodontic origin, then reattachment will usually occur, provided the lesion has not been longstanding. If resolution is only partial, then periodontal therapy will be required if a successful result is to be obtained. In cases of advanced periodontal disease, one or more roots may require resection after root canal therapy.

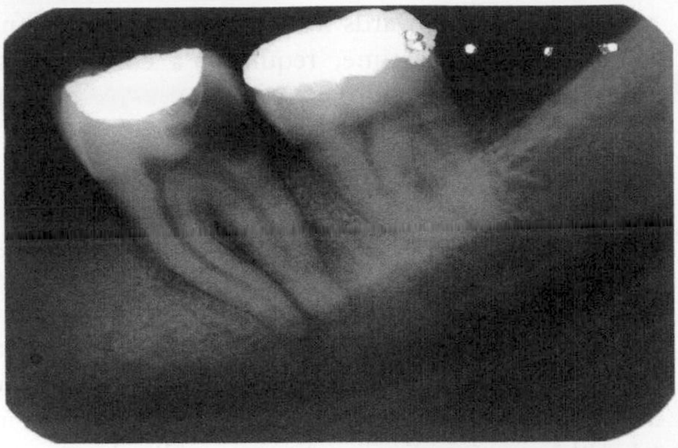

A

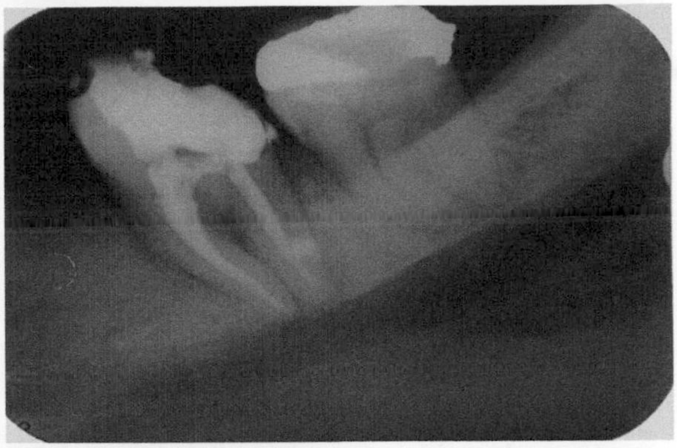

B

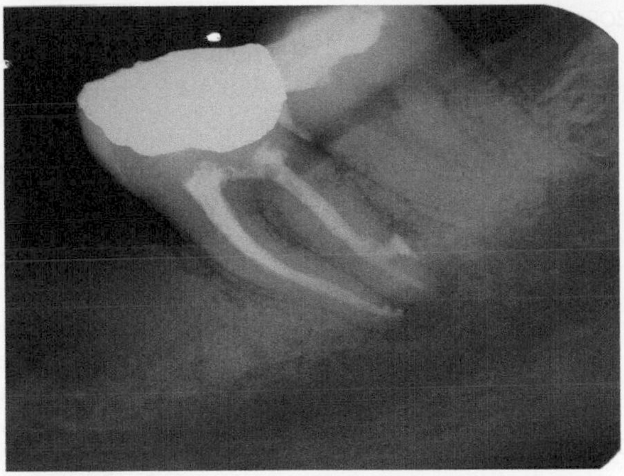

C

Figure 3.11 (A) Tooth can be restored and is therefore suitable for root canal therapy. (B) Caries removed and root canal therapy completed. (C) Follow-up 6 months after restoration.

Box 3.4 Some key aspects of endodontic diagnosis and case selection

- Diagnosis
  - — duplicate the patient's main complaint
- Treatment plan
  - — look at the tooth in the context of the rest of the patient's dentition
- Extract teeth that are:
  - — unrestorable
  - — have hopeless periodontal prognosis
  - — are cracked

Cracked teeth

This appears to be an increasing clinical problem.[3] Small cracks may be treatable, although communications through the floor of the pulp chamber or root canal usually result in tooth loss.

Re-root treatment

Re-root treatment is an increasing clinical problem and is considered more fully in Chapter 8.

Contraindications to treatment

General factors

The patient's medical history or general wellbeing may preclude treatment. If there is an indication for antibiotic cover then it should be given, as even if the instrumentation does not cause a bacteraemia, the placement of a rubber dam most likely will. Lack of patient interest or restricted opening may preclude endodontic treatment. Access to posterior teeth may be difficult, with a minimum of two fingers' opening being required. Remember that any degree of opening may reduce as the patient's jaw muscles become fatigued.

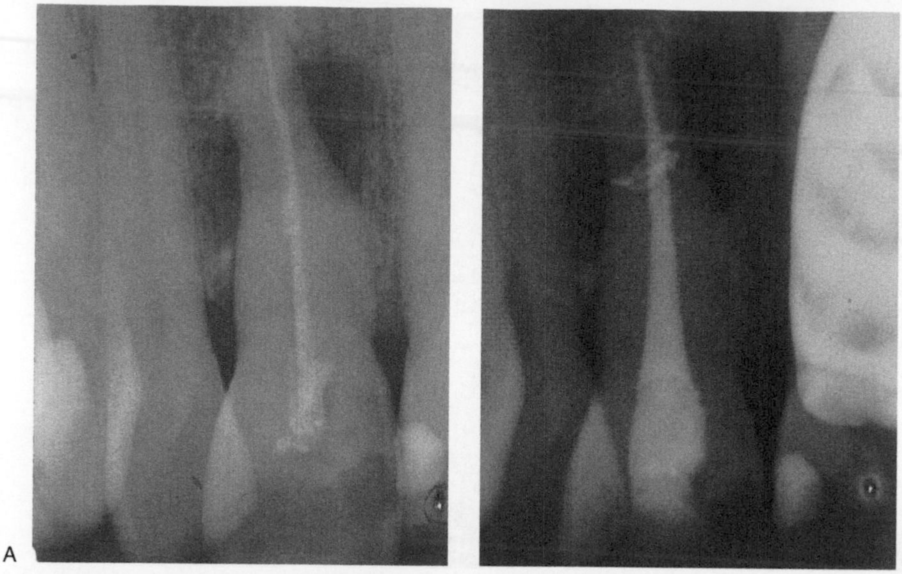

Figure 3.12 (A, B) Horizontal root fracture before and after treatment. Normally the tooth is only treated to the fracture line; however, in this case the apical portion was removed surgically as it was infected. Frequently root canal therapy is only required to the fracture line with the apical section being left undisturbed provided apical periodontitis is not present.

Restorative factors

The clinical examination may have revealed the tooth to be unrestorable, to be of little functional use or to have a hopeless periodontal prognosis. Such situations preclude root canal therapy. Other forms of pathology may be present, such as extensive internal or external resorption. Although internal resorption will cease once the pulp is removed, consideration must be made as to the strength of the remaining root in function.

Trauma

Root fractures may be present either horizontally (Fig. 3.12) or vertically (Fig. 3.13). Horizontal root fractures in the middle to apical third can have quite a good prognosis as the apical segment frequently remains vital, with root canal therapy only being necessary to the fracture line. Fractures involving the gingival crevice, however, rapidly become infected as there is a continuation of the fracture line and the periodontal space. This includes vertical root fractures and many oblique fractures resulting from trauma. The presence of a vertical root fracture may need to be confirmed by lifting a flap to allow direct inspection of the root surface.[4]

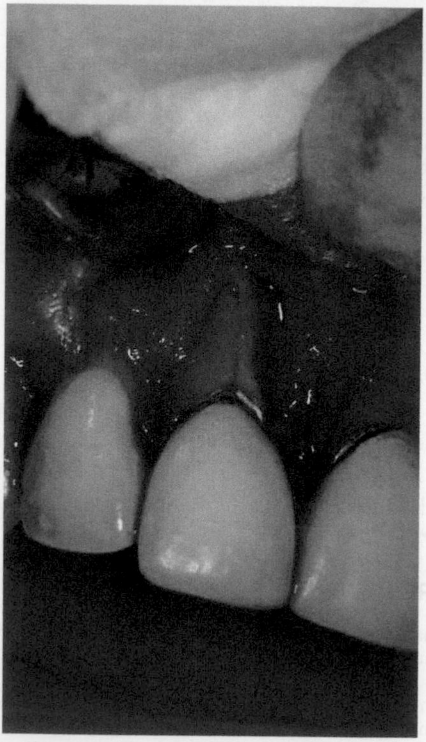

Figure 3.13 Vertical root fracture as revealed by direct inspection following raising of a flap.

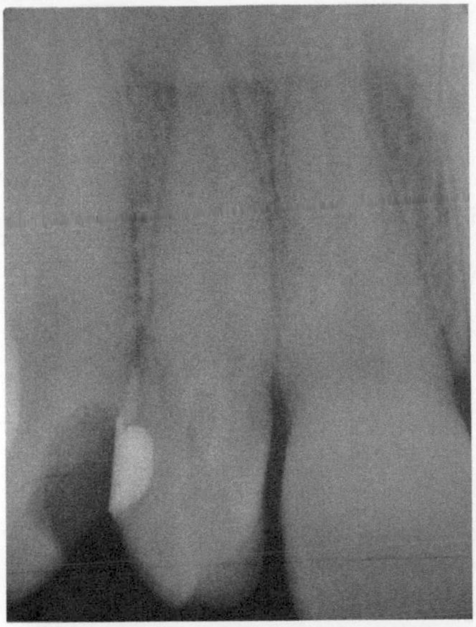

A

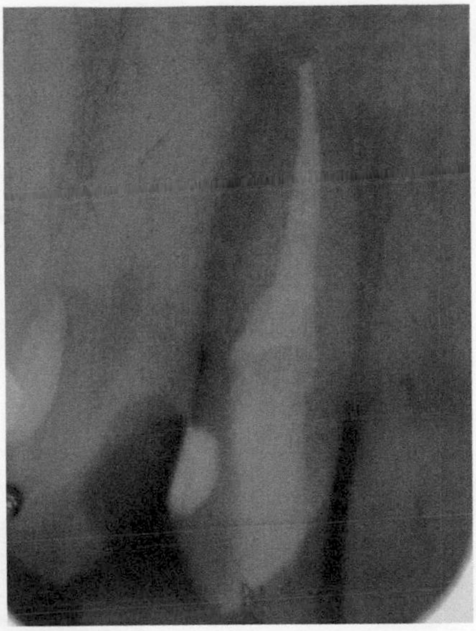

C

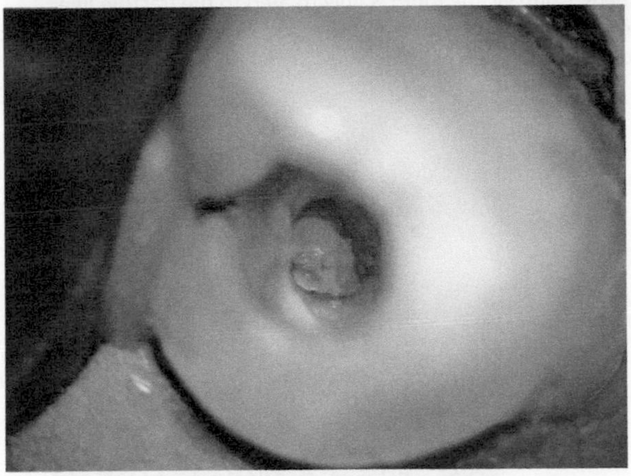

B

Figure 3.14 (A–C) Small dens in dente such as the one presented here may be treated endodontically; however, more involved ones may not respond, due to the presence of infection in the convoluted anatomy.

Complex internal or external anatomy

Other contraindications include anatomy that is too complex to treat. Such variations may be internal (dens in dente, Fig. 3.14) or external (root grooves). Palatal root grooves on upper incisors have a poor prognosis as again there is a continuum along the external aspect of the root which, like a root fracture, cannot be adequately cleaned and represents a constant nidus of infection.

REFERENCES

1. Hyman JJ, Cohen ME. The predictive value of endodontic diagnostic tests. Oral Surg Oral Med Oral Pathol 1984; 58: 343–346.
2. Chambers F. The role and method of pulp testing in oral diagnosis. Int Endod J 1982; 15: 1–15.
3. Cameron CE. The cracked tooth syndrome. Additional findings. J Am Dent Assoc 1976; 93: 971–975.
4. Pitts DL, Natkin E. Diagnosis and treatment of vertical root fractures. J Endod 1984; 9: 338–346.

4 Root canal anatomy and access

The anatomy of the root canal system is more complicated than has traditionally been taught. It has been shown by a number of techniques, from injecting vulcanite into the root canal system in the 1920s,[1] to recently introduced computerized tomography,[2] that the root canal system emanating from the pulp chamber is complex. It consists of lateral canals, accessory canals, fins and apical deltas as well as the main canal (Figs 4.1 and 4.2).

PULP CHAMBER

In general, the anatomy of the crown of the tooth is a projection of the cross-sectional outline of the pulp chamber with location of the canal orifice often being below the cusp tip or cingulum in posterior and anterior teeth, respectively. Obviously, if the tooth has a cast restoration then the anatomy will be altered and some care may be needed in locating the root canals. The dentine of the floor of the pulp chamber is often blue/grey in colour and is different from the walls. This knowledge can be usefully used as an aid in locating a root canal orifice. It is also possible to map the location of the orifi using grooves that are seen in the floor of the chamber, with orifi often being found along or at the junction of grooves.

Root canals

The main root canal is favourable to mechanical instrumentation but lateral canals, accessory canals and fins[3] can only be cleaned via chemical means, since it may be impossible to access these mechanically (Fig. 4.2).

Apical anatomy

The root canal terminates at the apical foramen (Fig. 4.3), where it emerges onto the external surface of the root up to 3 mm away from the anatomical apex.[4] The apical constriction represents the narrowest part of the root canal and is found slightly coronal to the apical foramen. The canal funnels out from the apical constriction to the apical foramen. The anatomy of the apical region has been analysed in a number of studies[5–7] and the apical constriction has been shown to be approximately 0.5 mm from the apical foramen. The diameter and configuration (Fig. 4.4)[5] of the apical foramen can also vary from 0.3 mm in a mandibular incisor to 0.6 mm in a mandibular molar. These research findings have clinical implications in establishing working length and width, including the use of electronic apex locators and will be discussed in subsequent chapters.

Classification of root canal morphology

There are two classification systems for assessing root canal morphology: that of Weine[8] and Vertucci.[9] Whilst the latter covers more detailed canal configuration, the Weine system is simpler and easier to apply clinically. The Weine classification is summarized in Box 4.1.

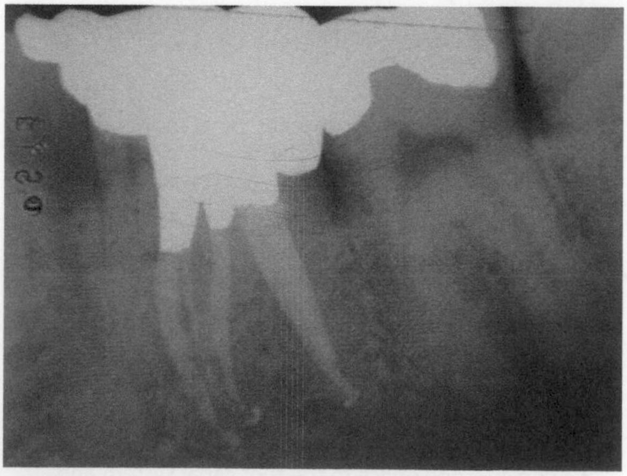

Figure 4.1 Postoperative radiograph of lower first molar showing complex anatomy in the mesial root and multiple apical foramina.

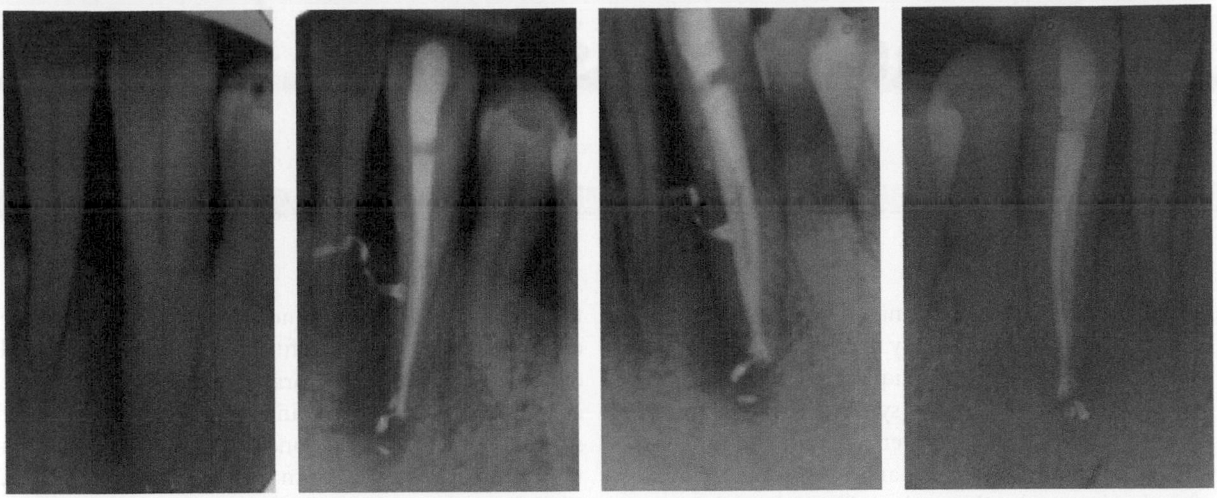

Figure 4.2 (A–D) Preoperative, post obturation and 6 month follow-up views of lower canine demonstrating lateral canals and apical delta.

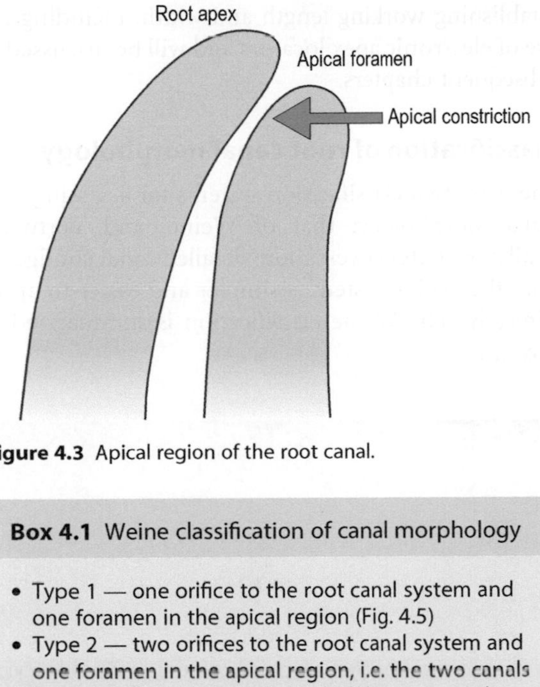

Figure 4.3 Apical region of the root canal.

Box 4.1 Weine classification of canal morphology

- Type 1 — one orifice to the root canal system and one foramen in the apical region (Fig. 4.5)
- Type 2 — two orifices to the root canal system and one foramen in the apical region, i.e. the two canals fuse, usually in the apical third of the root canal to give one canal in the apical region (Fig. 4.6)
- Type 3 — two orifices to the root canal system and two main foramina in the apical region, i.e. the two canals remain separate to the apical foramina (Fig. 4.7)
- Type 4 — one orifice to the root canal system and the canal divides to form two separate canals and foramina in the apical region (Fig. 4.8)

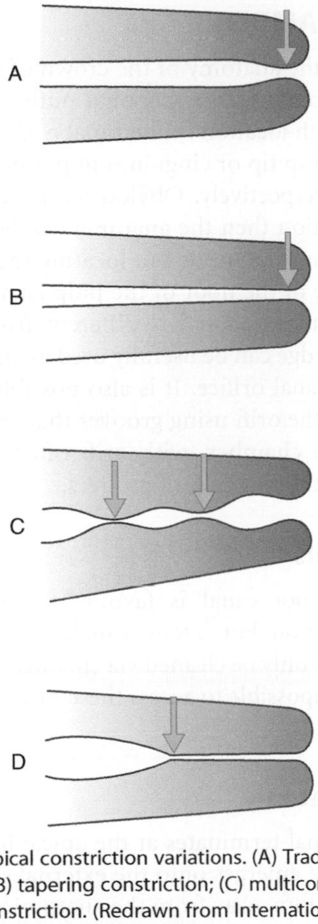

Figure 4.4 Apical constriction variations. (A) Traditional single constriction; (B) tapering constriction; (C) multiconstricted; (D) parallel constriction. (Redrawn from International Endodontic Journal, with permission.)

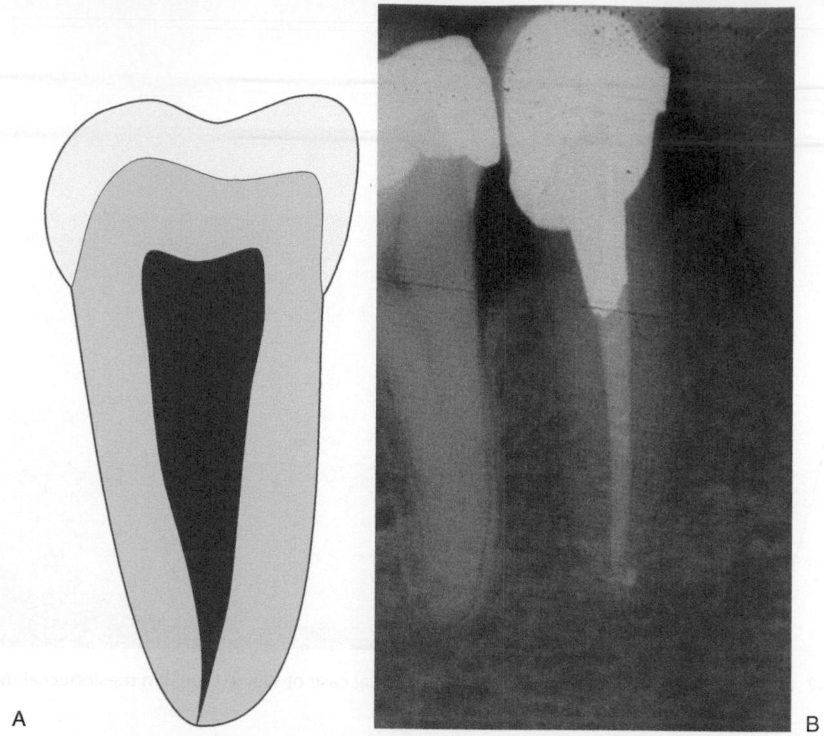

Figure 4.5 (A) Diagram of Weine type 1 anatomy. (B) Clinical case of Weine type 1.

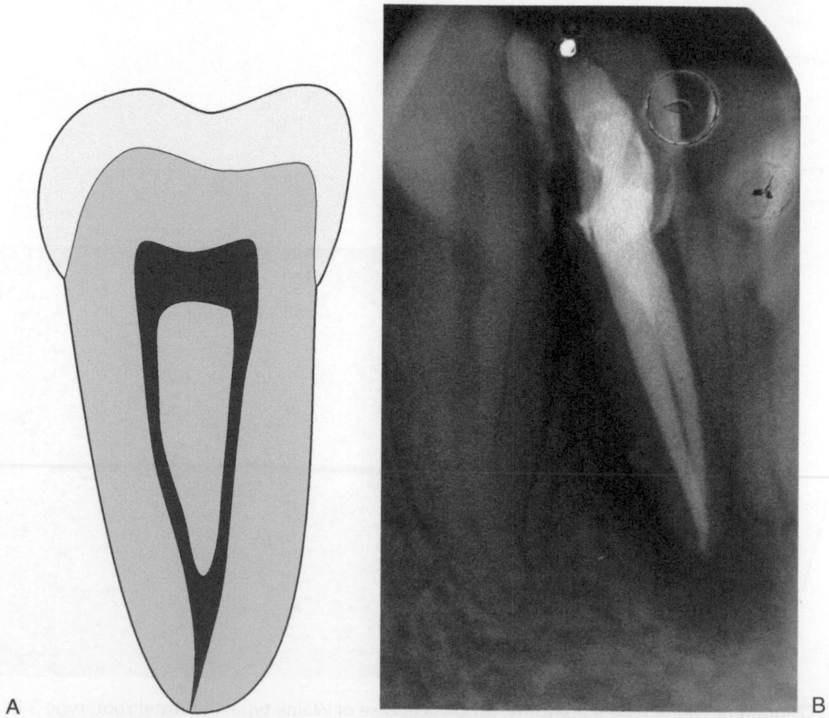

Figure 4.6 (A) Diagram of Weine type 2 anatomy. (B) Clinical case of Weine type 2.

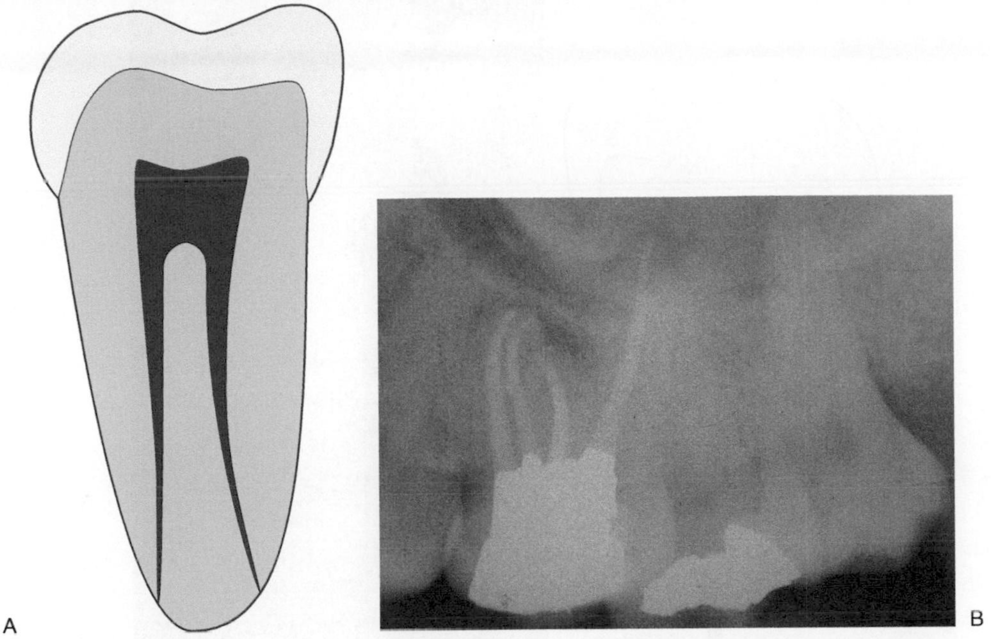

Figure 4.7 (A) Diagram of Weine type 3 anatomy. (B) Clinical case of Weine type 3 in mesiobuccal (MB) root.

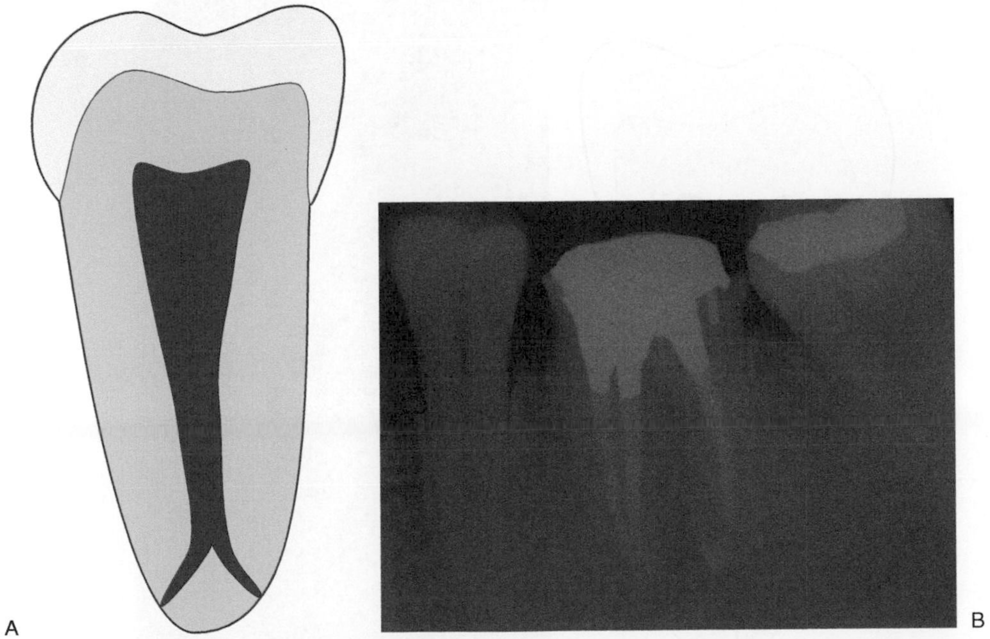

Figure 4.8 (A) Diagram of Weine type 4 anatomy. (B) Clinical case of Weine type 4 in distal root, type 3 in mesial root.

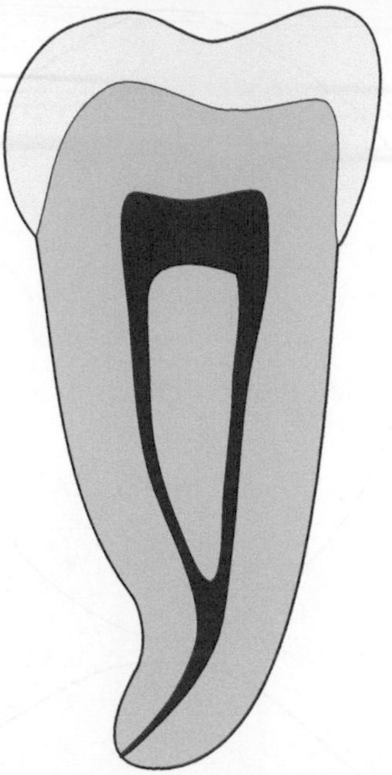

Figure 4.9 Type 2 anatomy in a lower molar mesial root. The buccal and lingual canals have S and single curves, respectively. This can be checked clinically by using two small files and evaluating their depth of penetration individually and together. It is advisable to treat the single curved canal as the main canal in such situations.

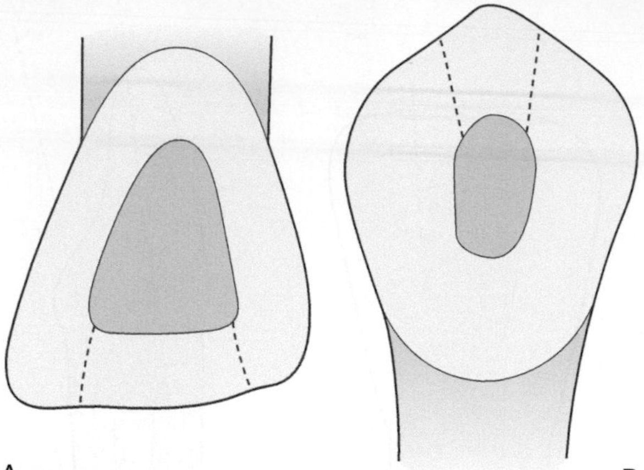

A B

Figure 4.10 Access cavity outline of (A) upper incisor and (B) upper/lower canine.

It is advantageous to establish the type of canal morphology as early in the procedure as possible, whilst being consistent with the principles of canal preparation. For example, knowing the morphology is a type 2 may prevent the operator from placing a rotary nickel titanium file unknowingly through an S-shaped aspect of a canal, thus reducing the risk of file breakage (Fig. 4.9).

ENDODONTIC ACCESS OPENINGS AND APPLIED ANATOMY

Incisor and canine teeth

The access cavities for maxillary central and lateral incisors are similar and generally triangular in shape (Fig. 4.10A). Access cavities for maxillary and mandibular canines are almost identical and more ovoid in shape (Fig. 4.10B).

Lower incisors

The root of these teeth is broad buccolingually, and narrow in the mesiodistal aspect. Nearly 50% of these teeth have two orifices to the root canal system, but the majority fuse in the apical third to give one canal in the apical region and one apical foramen, i.e. they are Weine type 2. Only 1.3% of these canal systems remain separate to the apical foramen, i.e. Weine type 3.[9,10] The two canals are found buccally and lingually and it is often the lingual canal that is more difficult to locate. In general, the access cavity should be extended towards the incisal edge and under the cingulum (Fig. 4.11).

Premolar teeth

Upper premolars

Commonly, first premolars have two roots and second premolars one. Normally the access cavity will be extended more buccolingually for two as opposed to single rooted premolar teeth (Fig. 4.12). Occasionally (5%), upper premolar teeth have three roots, two buccal and one palatal. Location of the orifices of the root canals in the buccal roots can be difficult, since they are often at the level of the crestal bone and care must be taken not to perforate the pulpal floor (Fig. 4.13).

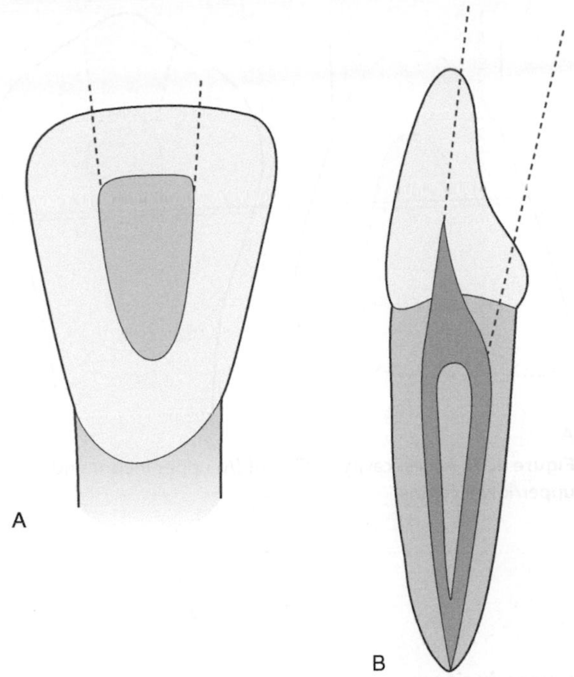

Figure 4.11 (A) Access cavity outline of lower incisor, showing applied anatomy (B).

Lower premolars

These teeth are probably the most common teeth in which to find the Weine type 4 morphology. Diagnostically, the preoperative radiograph is important, since the canal will be very broad in the coronal aspect of the tooth, and then 'disappears'. It is at this level that the canals usually divide (Fig. 4.14).

Upper molars

The maxillary molar access cavity outline is generally triangular in shape with the base to the buccal and the apex to the palatal. These teeth normally have three roots, the mesial and the distal being the buccal roots, and a palatal root. The first molar is generally larger than the second molar and this tooth is more likely to have fused roots. The mesial root of these teeth has two canals, although it is not always possible to locate them clinically. The second canal in this root is generally found in the area shown in Figure 4.15A and frequently requires extension of the access cavity outline into the mesial marginal ridge.

Four canals have been located in 93% of teeth for the first molar and 60% for the second molar.[11] The morphology of these root canal systems is usually

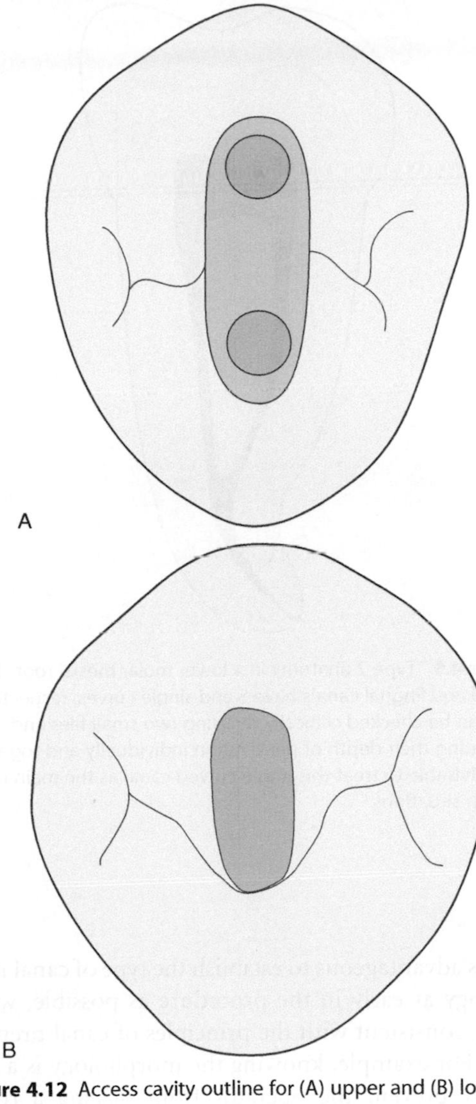

Figure 4.12 Access cavity outline for (A) upper and (B) lower premolar teeth.

Weine types 2 and 3, with type 4 seldom being found. Rarely, there are three canals to the mesial root of upper molars (Fig. 4.16).

Lower molars

The mandibular molar access cavity outline is more trapezoid in shape, with its base to the mesial and apex to the distal. These teeth generally have two roots, a mesial and a distal. Again, the first molar is larger than the second molar, and the latter is more likely to have fused roots. The mesial root generally has two root canals, with the canal morphology usually being

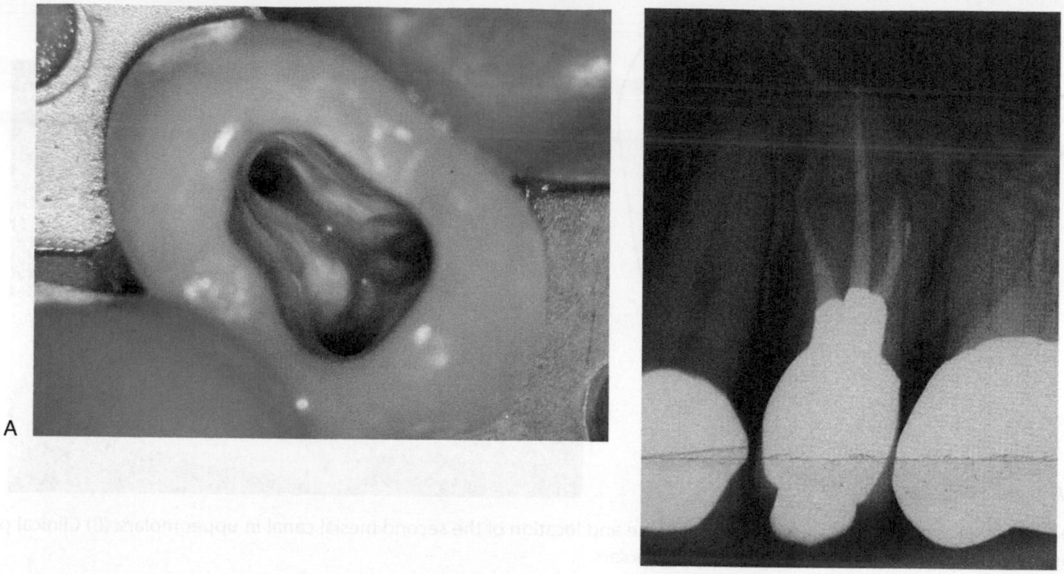

Figure 4.13 (A) Clinical picture and (B) radiograph of upper premolar with three canals.

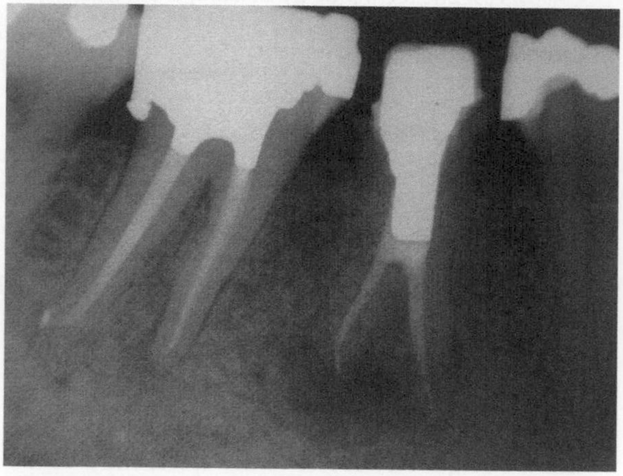

Figure 4.14 Lower premolar indicating Weine type 4 anatomy.

Weine type 2 or 3. The distal root has one canal in 75% of cases, and two in 25%. An important diagnostic feature is the location of the distal orifice in relation to the mid-point of the tooth on the mesiodistal axis (Fig. 4.17).

If the orifice lies on this line then there will be one distal canal; if it does not, then there will be a second orifice to locate on the opposite side of the tooth. The morphology of the distal canal can be Weine type 2, 3 or 4. In the last case it is important to carry out a thorough exploration of the sub-orifice region before eliminating the possibility of a type 4 and confirming a type 1 canal system. It should also be noted that, with the improved illumination and magnification available with operating microscopes, a third canal is now being located more frequently in the mesial root (Fig. 4.18).

Rubber dam

The use of rubber dam is mandatory in endodontic therapy, being fundamental to aseptic practice. Frequently the use of dam is linked to preventing inhalation or swallowing of instruments. Clearly this is an important feature of its use; however, it is timely, with the advent of an increased number of instrumentation systems where files are held in a handpiece, to reinforce the biological reasons for using rubber dam.

The dam is a thin sheet of rubber placed around the tooth and acts as a barrier. This sheet may be held in place using a clamp or occasionally thin pieces of rubber between the teeth. Many examples of rubber dam isolation may be found in this text; normally a simple technique is all that is required when isolating only a single tooth. Occasionally it may be necessary to use a slit dam technique which involves placement

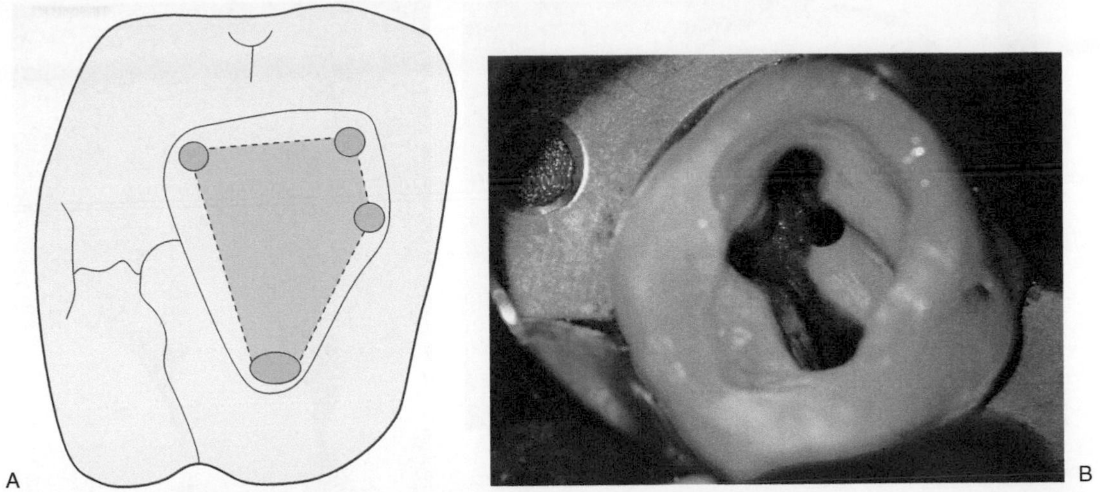

Figure 4.15 (A) Diagram showing access cavity outline and location of the second mesial canal in upper molars. (B) Clinical picture of location of second canal in the mesial root of upper molars.

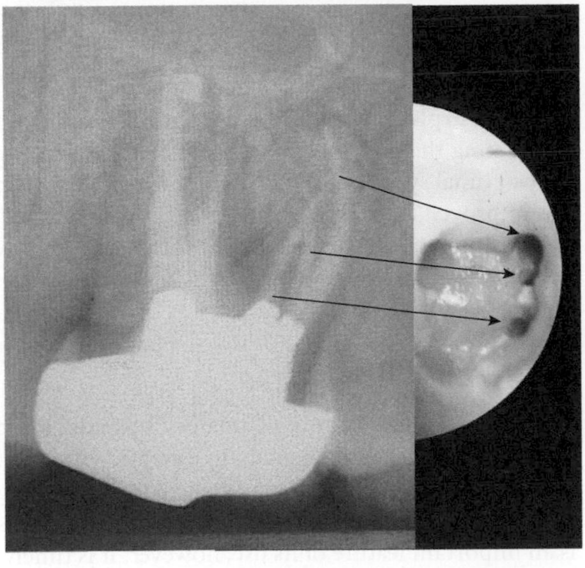

Figure 4.16 Radiograph and clinical photograph of three mesial canal orifi in an upper molar.

of more than one tooth through the dam. In such situations complete isolation may be more challenging. It is important that the seal is checked following all dam placements; if it is found to be inadequate, a ring of hard setting $Ca(OH)_2$ cement or Oroseal may be placed around the tooth to preclude leakage of saliva. Some advantages of rubber dam isolation are outlined in Box 4.2.

Box 4.2 Some advantages of rubber dam isolation

- Allows aseptic technique by isolating tooth from saliva
- Contains antimicrobial irrigants
- Improves visibility
- Protects soft tissues
- Reduces medicolegal liability

Access

The principles of gaining access to the root canal system are as follows:

- Remove the entire contents of the pulp chamber
- Allow inspection of all of the pulp chamber floor
- Allow straight line access to the apical third of the root canal.

The access cavity should be prepared with these objectives in mind and also should:

- remove the entire roof of the pulp chamber
- allow visualization of all root canal orifices
- be dynamic, i.e. should be enlarged if straight line access to all canals cannot be obtained via the initial cavity
- have convergent walls in an apical direction to support the temporary dressing (and reduce the risk of leakage).

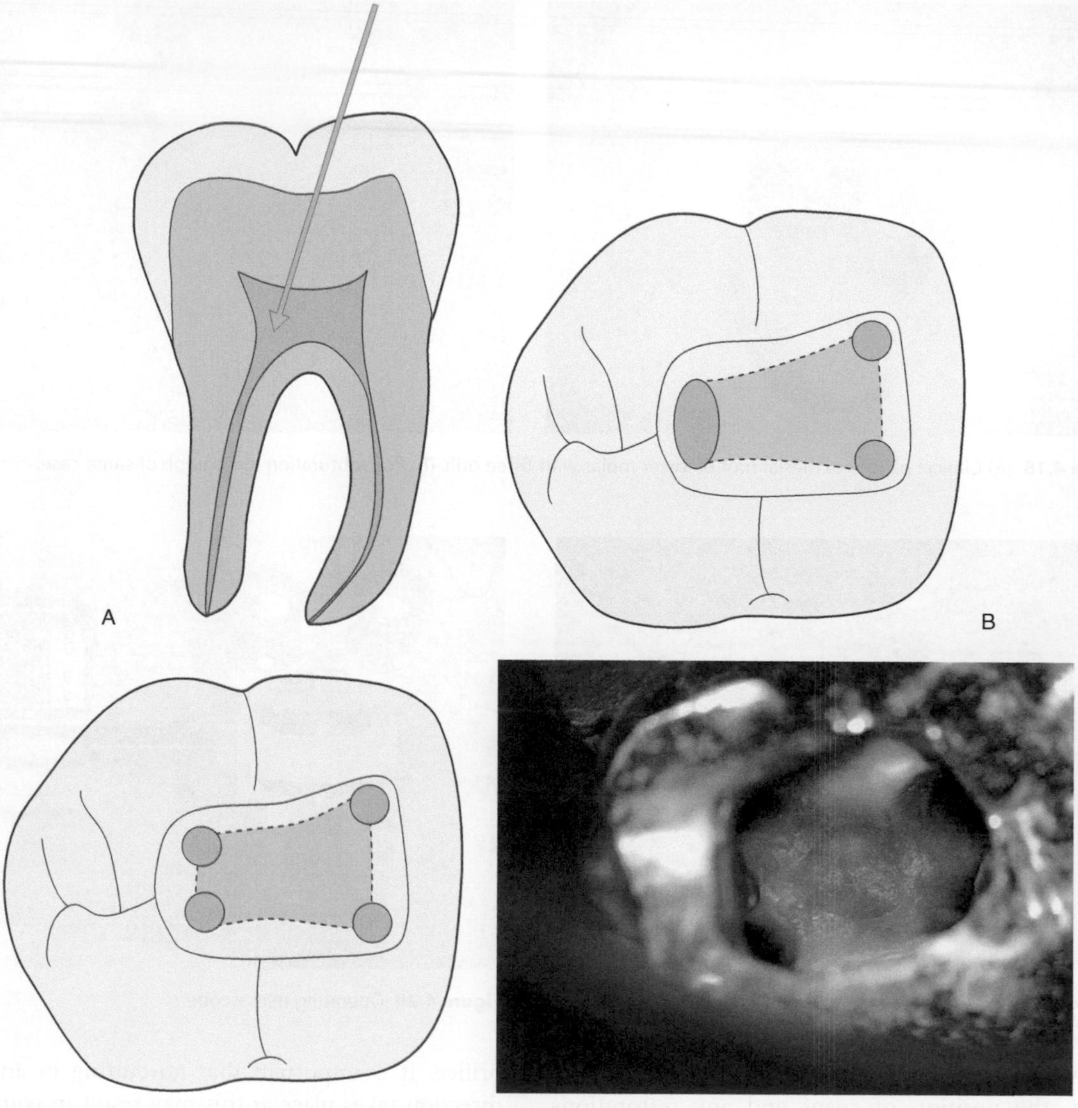

Figure 4.17 Canal anatomy of distal root in lower molars. (A) Initial entry for the distal may normally be made in the mid mesial groove region. (B, C) show occlusal outline with the usual variants in anatomy. (D) Clinical picture of lower molar with two canals in the distal root.

Loupes (Fig. 4.19) and the operating microscope (Fig. 4.20) afford excellent visibility, and have been shown to aid detection of additional root canals. It has been demonstrated[12] that magnification increases the incidence of canal location, with loupes being responsible for the largest increase in detection. However, the detail of more difficult canal location requires a knowledge of not only where to look but also what to look for, especially when using the operating microscope; such skills are only developed through extensive use. Figure 4.21 shows the range of magnification available with the operating microscope which also has the additional benefit of improved posture and consequent reduction in operator back pain (Fig. 4.22).

CLINICAL PROCEDURE IN ACCESS CAVITY PREPARATION

It is essential to have good preoperative radiographs prior to commencing access cavity preparation. Ideally this will include two angles: straight-on and distal angle for molar teeth and straight-on and mesial angle

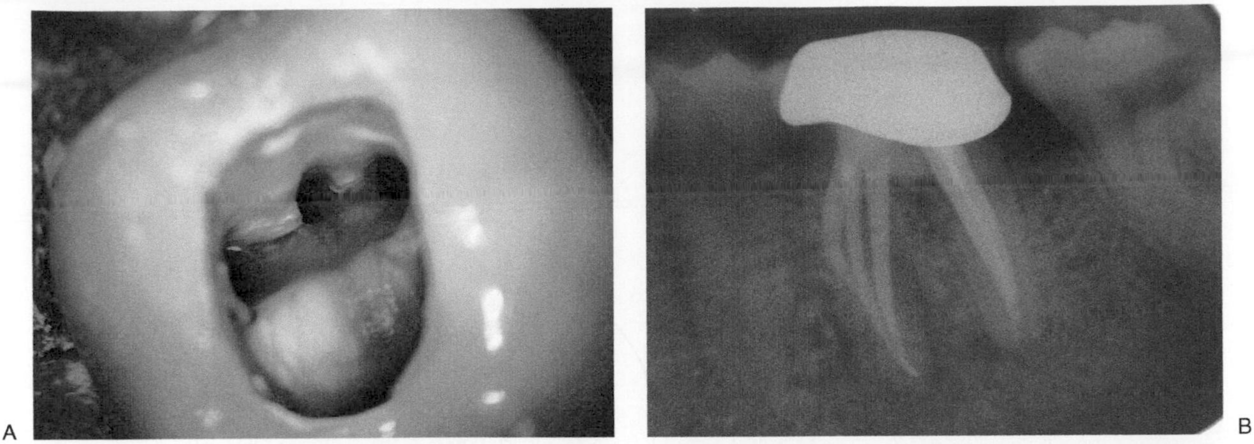

Figure 4.18 (A) Clinical picture of mesial root of lower molar with three orifi. (B) Post-obturation radiograph of same case.

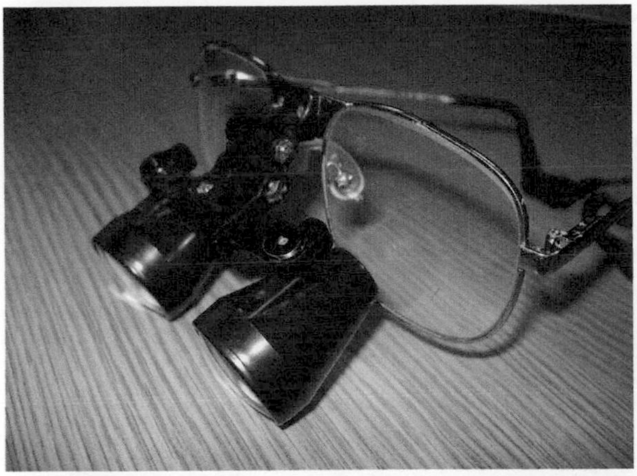

Figure 4.19 Loupes.

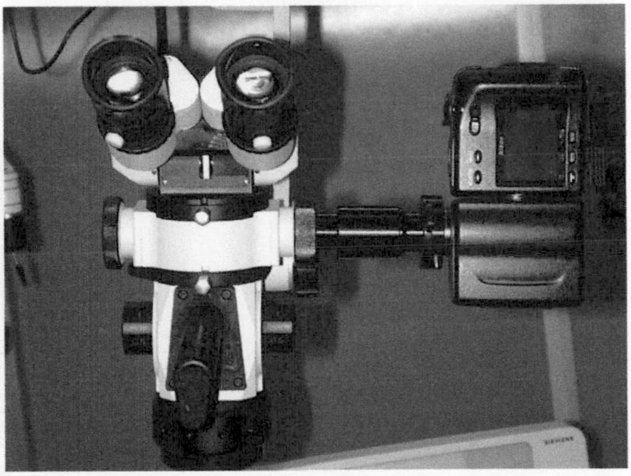

Figure 4.20 Operating microscope.

for premolar and anterior teeth. The angulation of the tooth, the position of cusps and any restorations should be noted. Palpation of the buccal and, where appropriate, lingual tissues will help in determining the position and angulation of the root. Ideally the access cavity should be prepared under rubber dam, but there are circumstances (e.g. difficult tooth angulation) where it may be advisable to gain initial access to the pulp chamber prior to dam placement. In these circumstances it is important to prevent damage to the tooth in the attempt to locate the pulp chamber and root canal orifice.

Initial entry is made through the enamel or restorative material with a high-speed bur. Once the bur has entered the pulp chamber, a safe-ended bur is used to flare out the access preparation to locate the root canal orifice. It is important that no cutting in an apical direction takes place as this may result in gouging of the pulp chamber floor or perforation. Once this initial access preparation has been completed, the canal orifices are located with an endodontic explorer such as DG16 (Fig. 4.23). When the canal orifices have been located, the initial access cavity may need to be refined to allow adequate access to the root canal of coronal shaping instruments. Further refinements to the outline of the access cavity may be required as one of the principles of good access preparation is to allow straight line access to the apical third of the root canal system. It should be appreciated that the outline of the access cavity is being constantly refined from its initial outline to allow optimum access to the root canal system.

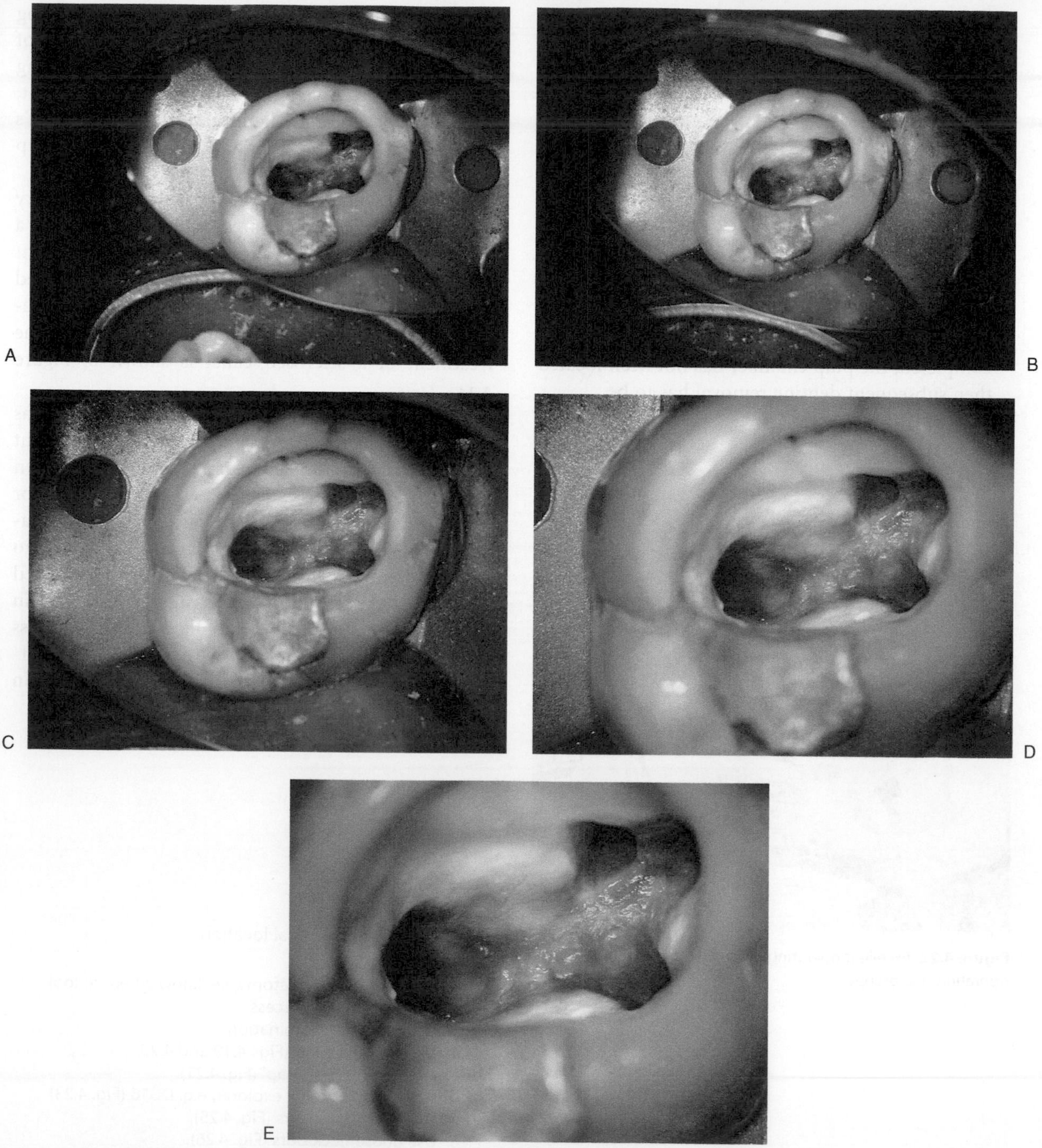

Figure 4.21 Magnification through the microscope; note furcal canal. (A) 3.5× magnification; (B) 6× magnification; (C) 8× magnification; (D) 12× magnification; (E) 16× magnification.

Where the pulp chamber appears sclerosed on the preoperative radiograph, additional precautions are required:

- The initial preparation bur should be lined up against the preoperative radiograph to make an assessment of pulp chamber floor depth and avoid perforation of the pulp chamber floor.
- If there is an area of partial sclerosis the access cavity should initially be directed away from this area so that the chances of locating the pulp chamber are increased.
- If, after the initial access preparation has been completed, the pulp chamber has not been located then subsequent dentine removal has to be completed with caution.

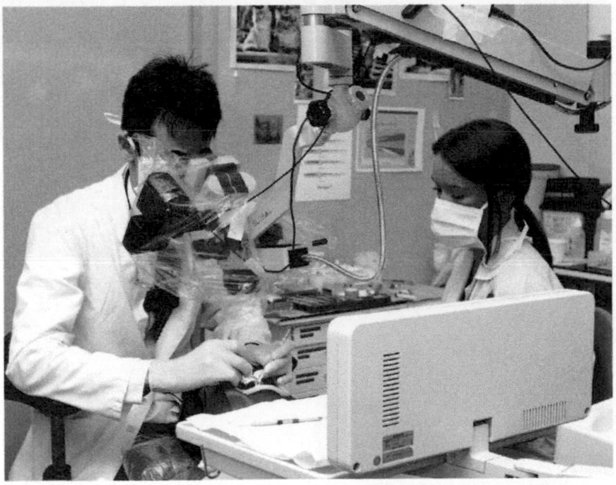

Figure 4.22 Excellent operating posture afforded by the operating microscope.

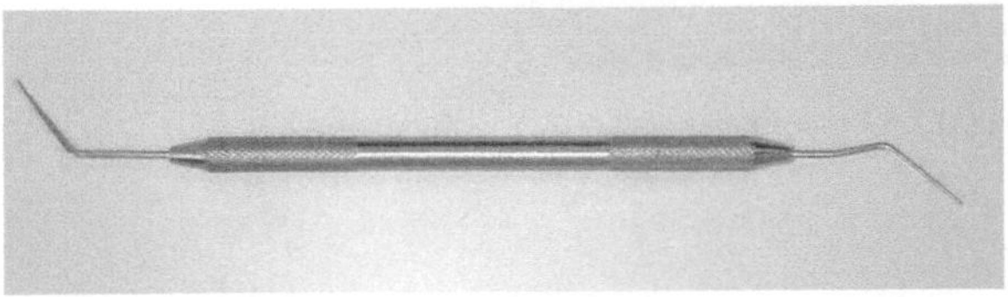

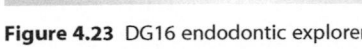

Figure 4.23 DG16 endodontic explorer.

It is advisable to continue preparation with long shank, slow-speed burs or ultrasonic tips. Both of these instruments have the advantage that the long shank allows direct vision of the tip of the instrument, i.e. both the head of the handpiece and the operator's fingers do not impede vision of the small cutting tip of the instrument.

In the case of sclerosed canals, it may be necessary to place a small file in the area of the canal and take a radiograph to check for alignment of the instrument related to the canal. This procedure may be repeated as instrumentation progresses apically. The management location, opening and final radiograph of the treatment of a sclerosed canal is shown in Figure 4.24.

Cuspal reduction may be considered on occasion as an adjunct to canal location as this allows more light into the chamber. Due consideration should be taken in regard to how this is performed as most posterior teeth require some form of cast cusp covered restoration following endodontic therapy. It is better to remove dentine, which will ultimately be removed during tooth preparation for a casting, at this stage in the endodontic procedure, and allow adequate access to all the root canals rather than compromise treatment. Some hints for canal location are outlined in Box 4.3.

Box 4.3 Hints for canal location

1. Know the tooth anatomy, i.e. know where to look
2. Create adequate access
3. Use adequate illumination
4. Use magnification (Figs 4.19 and 4.20)
5. Use the 'dentine map' (Fig. 4.21).
6. Use an endodontic explorer, e.g. DG16 (Fig. 4.23)
7. Use long shank burs (Fig. 4.25).
8. Use goose neck burs (Fig. 4.26).
9. Use ultrasonics (Fig. 4.27).
10. Use micro-openers and small files (Fig. 4.28)
11. Transillumination (Fig. 4.29).
12. Use a dye (Fig. 4.30).
13. Bubbles from hypochlorite (Fig. 4.31).

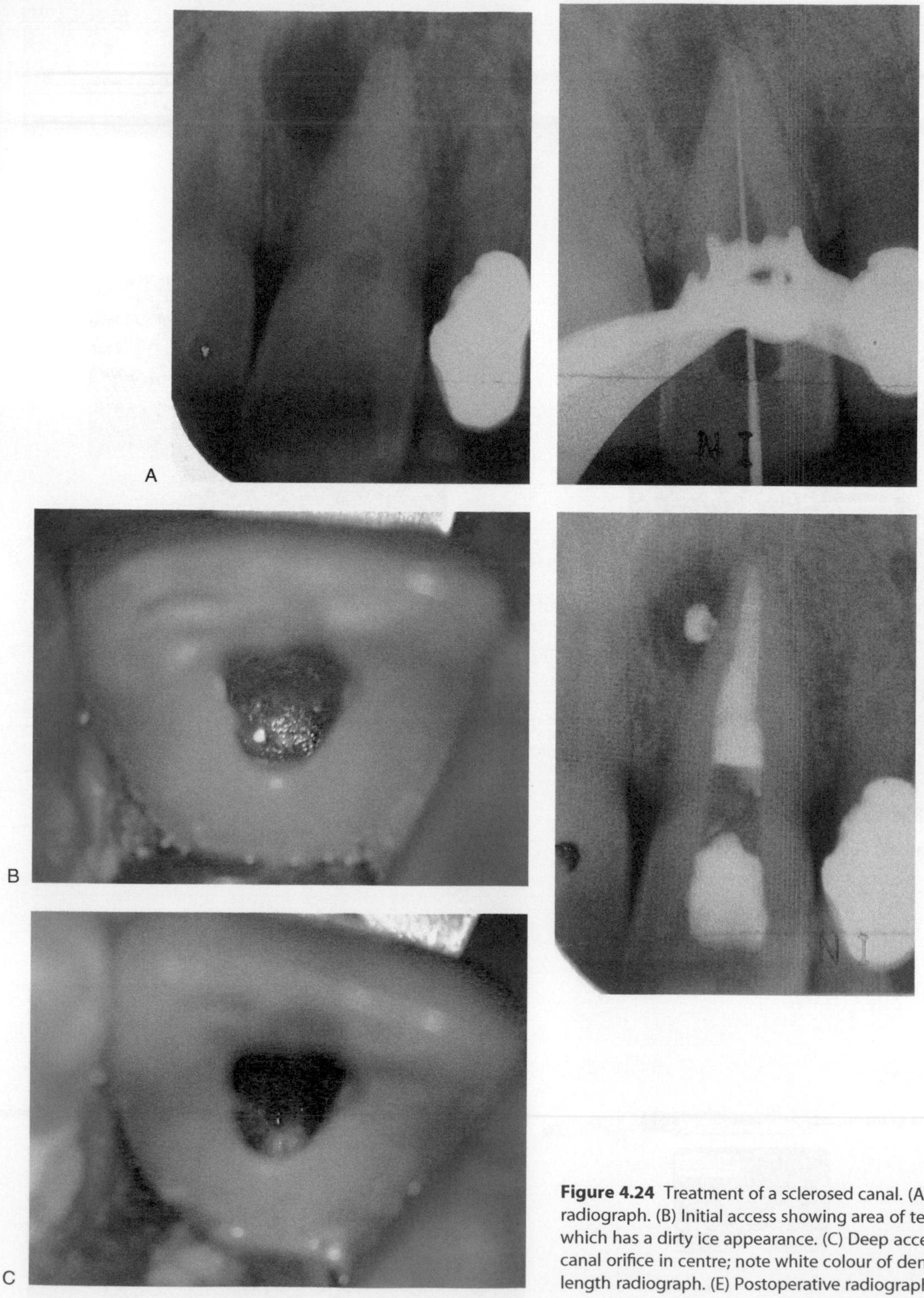

Figure 4.24 Treatment of a sclerosed canal. (A) Preoperative radiograph. (B) Initial access showing area of tertiary dentine which has a dirty ice appearance. (C) Deep access showing canal orifice in centre; note white colour of dentine. (D) Working length radiograph. (E) Postoperative radiograph.

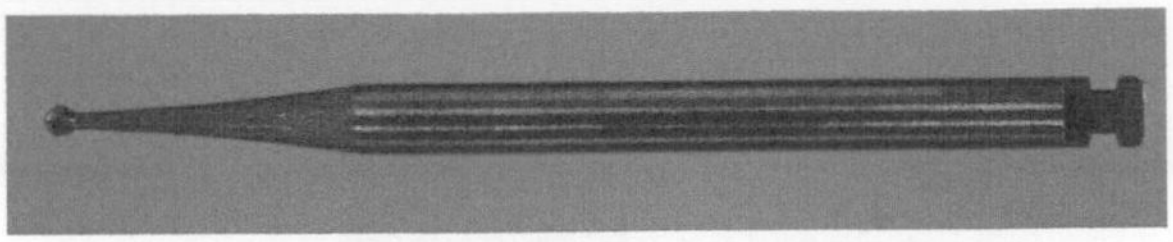

Figure 4.25 Long shank burs.

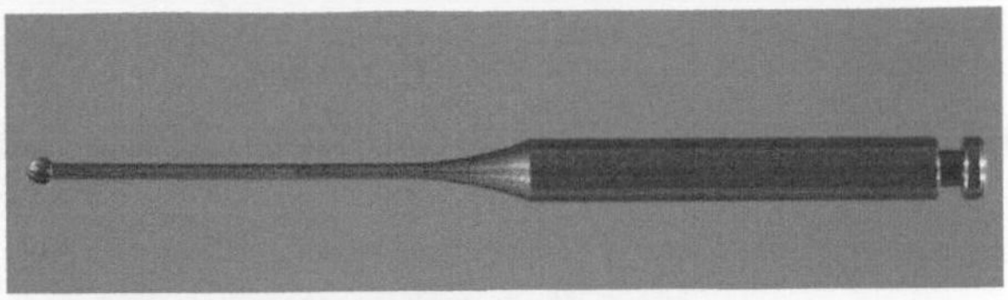

Figure 4.26 Goose neck burs.

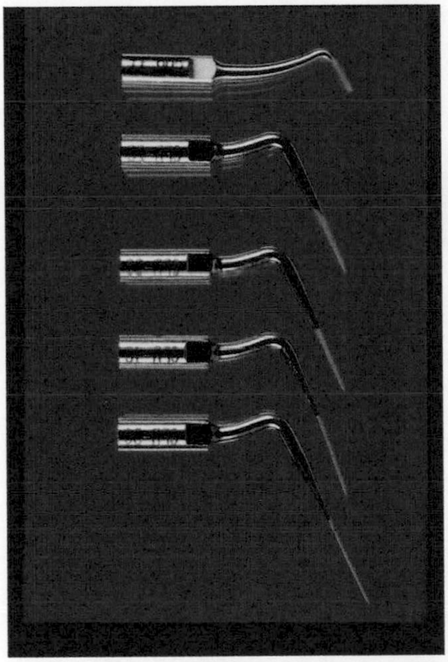

Figure 4.27 Ultrasonic tips used in removing dentine to locate canals.

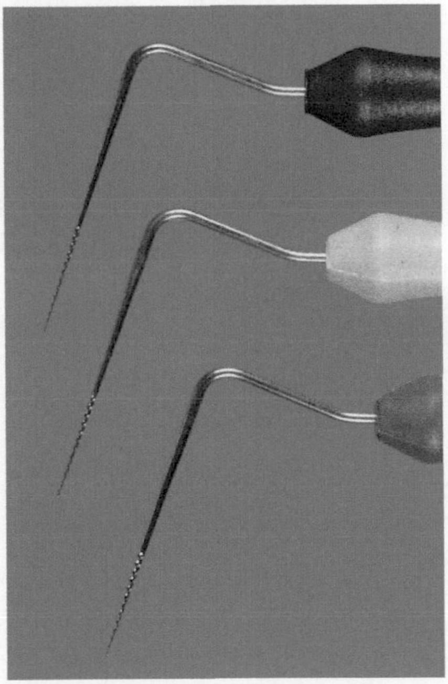

Figure 4.28 Micro-openers.

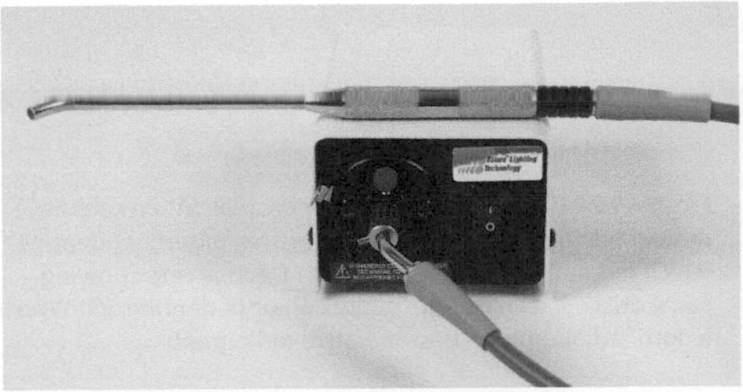

A

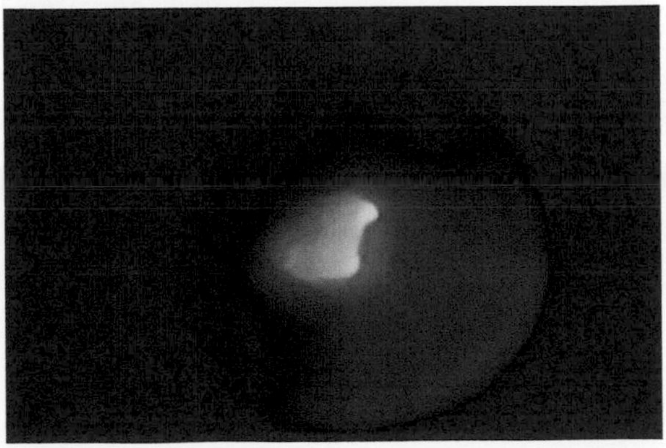

B

Figure 4.29 Transillumination of a tooth to aid canal location. (A) Illuminator; (B) view through microscope.

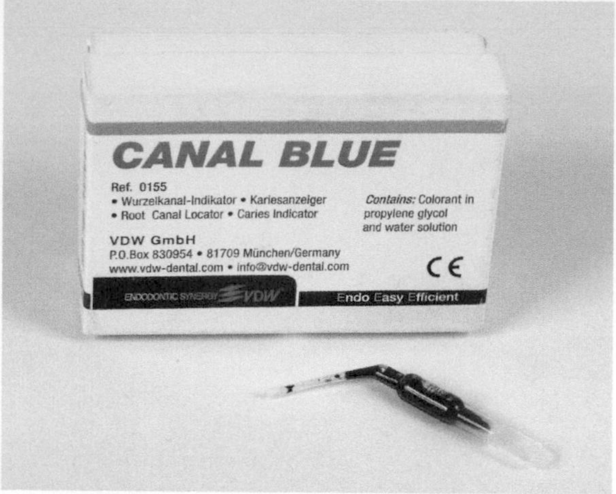

Figure 4.30 Dye used to aid location of a root canal.

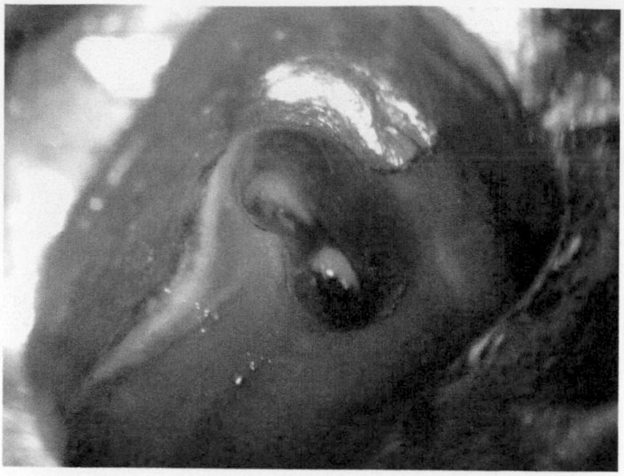

Figure 4.31 Mesial root of lower molar showing hypochlorite bubbles.

REFERENCES

1. Hess W, Zurcher E. The anatomy of the root canals of the teeth of the permanent and deciduous dentitions. New York: W. Wood and Co, 1925.
2. Peters OA, Laib A, Rüegsegger P, Barbakow F. Three dimensional analysis of root canal geometry using high resolution computed tomography. J Dent Res 2000; 79: 1405–1409.
3. De Deus Horizonte QD. Frequency, location and direction of lateral, secondary and accessory canals. J Endod 1975; 1: 361–366.
4. Kuttler Y. Microscopic investigation of root apexes. J Am Dent Assoc 1955; 50: 544–552.
5. Dummmer PMH, McGinn JH, Rees DG. The position and topography of the apical canal constriction and apical foramen. Int Endod J 1984; 17: 192–198.
6. Green D. A stereo-binocular microscope study of the root apices and surrounding areas of 100 mandibular molars. Oral Surg Oral Med Oral Pathol 1955; 8: 1298–1304.
7. Green D. A stereomicroscopic study of the root apices of 400 maxillary and mandibular anterior teeth. Oral Surg Oral Med Oral Pathol 1956; 9: 1224–1232.
8. Weine FS. Endodontic therapy, 5th edn. St Louis: Mosby, 1996: 243–244.
9. Vertucci FJ. Root canal anatomy of the human permanent teeth. Oral Surgery 1984; 58: 589–599.
10. Benjamin KA, Dowson J. Incidence of two root canals in human mandibular incisor teeth. Oral Surgery 1974; 38: 122–126.
11. Stropko JJ. Canal morphology of maxillary molars: clinical observations of canal configurations. J Endod 2000; 25: 446–450.
12. Buhrley LJ, Barrows MJ, BeGole EA, Wencus CS. Effect of magnification on locating the MB2 in maxillary molars. J Endod 2002; 28: 324–327.

5 Root canal preparation — objectives and instruments

OBJECTIVES

Root canal preparation is an essential step in endodontic treatment which aims to clean (debride and disinfect) the root canal system, create a shape that can be sealed from reinfection and leave sufficient tooth structure for the placement of a definitive final restoration. Cleaning and shaping are not separate events, as shaping removes infected dentine whilst creating space for the delivery of antibacterial agents such as irrigating solutions and intervisit dressing materials. Cleaning and shaping of root canals is achieved using both hand and rotary instruments and, most importantly, irrigating solutions. Modern preparation techniques can shape many canals rapidly; however, the complex nature of root canal systems means hand instruments still play an important role in exploring and finishing canal preparation, whilst irrigating solutions are essential for optimum cleaning.

One of the main controversies within endodontics[1] is where to finish the apical preparation, particularly in vital, compared with infected, cases. Studies[2,3] show that the location of the foramen varies from 0 to 3 mm from the anatomic apex. Much traditional teaching has centred around instrumenting to 1–2 mm short of the radiographic apex, as clinical studies have shown a 95% success rate in vital cases with this technique.[4] This can be explained by the position of the apical foramen and the natural healing process forming cementum-like tissue where some millimetres of the apical pulp tissue remain, following an aseptically performed partial pulpectomy.[5]

The necrotic infected pulp presents a different problem, however, as a result of possible bacterial presence at the apical foramen[6,7] and an understanding that the presence of apical periodontitis is associated with a reduced prognosis.[4,8] Ideally, the entire root canal should be instrumented in infected cases as it has been shown that in teeth/roots with apical periodontitis a millimetre loss in working length increased the chance of treatment failure by 14%,[9] and it is unlikely that antimicrobial agents will kill microbes in the apical portion of the root canal without adjunctive mechanical cleaning which may also help disperse the irrigant. The management of pulpitis with minimal infection may be left to personal preference as clinical experience shows that both instrumenting the entire root canal and slightly short have a favourable outcome.

Cleaning and shaping

Cleaning and shaping have both biological and mechanical objectives. The biological objectives of cleaning are to debride and disinfect the root canal system. This includes the removal of bacteria, related irritants and any organic material from the root canal system that may serve as a substrate for remaining bacteria and result in periradicular inflammation. In practice, this is achieved progressively through instrumentation, irrigation and intervisit dressing without the use of highly toxic medicaments. Mechanical preparation debrides the main root canal, but other parts of the root canal system, such as branches and isthmi, remain untouched. These areas may contain bacteria which can occasionally be reached by small files but, normally, intracanal irrigating solutions and medicaments provide disinfection in these areas. Shaping should be tailored to each individual root canal as all have their own specific internal and external anatomy, varying in length, curvature, cross-sectional diameter and profile. Cleaning and shaping is also a balance in regard to the amount of tooth substance left; it should not damage or weaken the root through overzealous apical or lateral preparation.

Cleaning and shaping of root canals is a natural continuation of access cavity preparation and canal identification, and aims to progressively decrease the bacterial infection within the tooth. It is essential that all caries is removed and the crown restored to allow rubber dam isolation and ensure a four-walled access cavity to contain irrigating solutions. The biological

objectives of canal preparation have been described by Schilder[10] and are listed in Box 5.1.

The mechanical objectives of canal preparation have been described by Schilder[10] and are listed in Box 5.2. These five mechanical objectives are now frequently referred to as four: continuously tapering preparation, original anatomy maintained, apical foramen in its original position and foramen as small as practical.

Root canal preparation emphasizes the creation of a continuously tapering shape from coronal to apical, appropriate to the individual root, using instruments large to small or greater to lesser taper, as discussed later. Modern preparation techniques have simplified the creation of this shape; however, certain canal forms, such as internal resorption, preclude its production, as to do so would grossly weaken the tooth. Tooth roots are infinitely variable in their anatomy, with some being oval coronally and more round apically, whereas others may be round along most of their length. No attempt is made to render the full length of every canal round as this would weaken oval roots unnecessarily or create a lateral perforation. In oval or dumb-bell shaped roots it is necessary to direct instruments laterally if the correct shape is to be achieved. The coronal regions of the root canal are normally more infected than the apical, thus preparing the root canal crown-down removes infected dentine and tissue remnants as they are encountered and creates shape/space to allow the deeper penetration of irrigating solutions and placement of intervisit dressing materials. Crown-down preparation also reduces the likelihood of apical extrusion of infected debris which, together with incomplete debridement, can be a cause of post-treatment pain in endodontics.[11]

Box 5.1 Biological objectives of canal preparation

1. Confine instrumentation to the root canals themselves. Do not routinely instrument bone or periapical lesions.
2. Beware of forcing necrotic material beyond the foramen during canal preparation.
3. Remove all tissue scrupulously from the root canal system.
4. Try to complete the cleaning and shaping of single canalled teeth in one visit and, whenever possible, to prepare multicanalled teeth one at a time.
5. Create sufficient space during canal enlargement to receive intracanal medicaments and to accommodate small amounts of periapical exudates should subclinical inflammation follow canal preparation.

After Schilder.[10]

Box 5.2 Mechanical objectives of canal preparation

1. The root canal preparation should develop a continuously tapering funnel from the root apex to the coronal access cavity.
2. In compliance with the above principle, the cross-sectional diameter of the preparation should be narrower at every point apically, and wider at each point as the access cavity is approached.
3. Unlike funnels of simple geometric design, this root canal preparation should occupy not only three planes, but as many as are presented by the root and root canal under treatment, i.e. the root canal should flow with the shape of the original canal.
4. The apical foramen should remain in its original spatial relationship both to the bone and to the root surface.
5. The apical opening should be kept as small as is practical in all cases.

After Schilder.[10]

Straight line access

Creation of straight line access, by removing coronal dentine overhangs in a controlled way, influences the forces a file exerts on the canal wall in the apical region (Fig. 5.1). This planned procedure helps to reduce

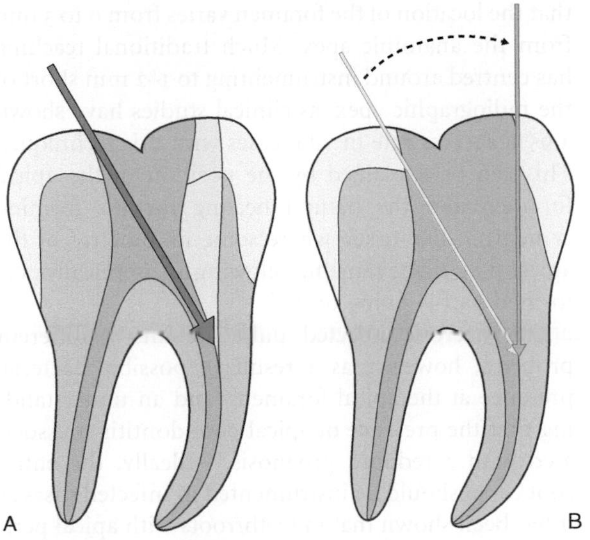

Figure 5.1 Access cavity (A) before and (B) after straight line access has been established.

inadvertent dentine removal in the mid root and apical areas which results from instruments, especially larger ones, trying to straighten. Uncontrolled mid root and apical removal of dentine away from the main canal can result in the final preparation not containing the original canal, weakening of the root and risk of perforation. This is especially important in curved canals, where files may remove more dentine along the inner furcal side as opposed to the outer canal wall, in the mid root area. An understanding of this concept is essential to ensure enlargement of curved canals is limited and instruments are directed away from the danger areas to avoid strip perforation (Fig. 5.2). In the apical region of the canal, dentine removal occurs more on the outer wall and can result in ledge formation or perforation in this area.

Preparation problems

It is important to prevent blockage and maintain a pathway for small instruments to follow in order that the continuously tapering preparation can be ensured along the full length of the canal. The interactions between instrument and dentine removal become more involved as canal complexity (such as S-shaped and severely curved root canals) increases. Frequently such cases can only be managed by using small files in a gentle push–pull manner if the natural anatomy and flow of the preparation are to be maintained (Fig. 5.3). The anatomy of an individual canal and the skill and patience of the operator therefore remain more important variables than the types of instrument used.

Many preparation problems occur due to mismanagement of the apical third of the root canal through

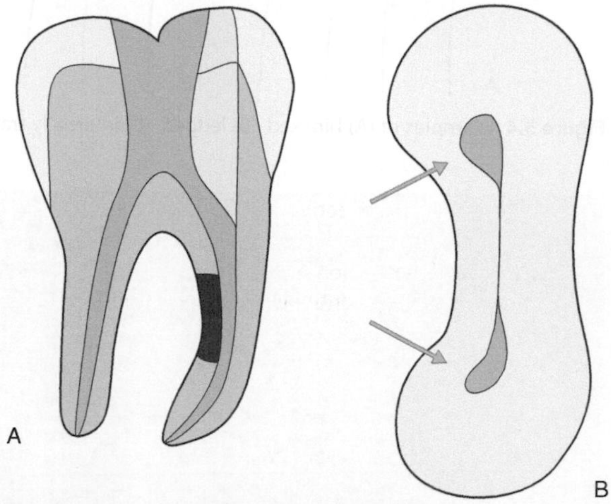

Figure 5.2 (A) Danger zone (red) on the inner side of root. (B) Strip perforation, in the area indicated by arrows, is a possibility, especially on the furcal side of curved roots.

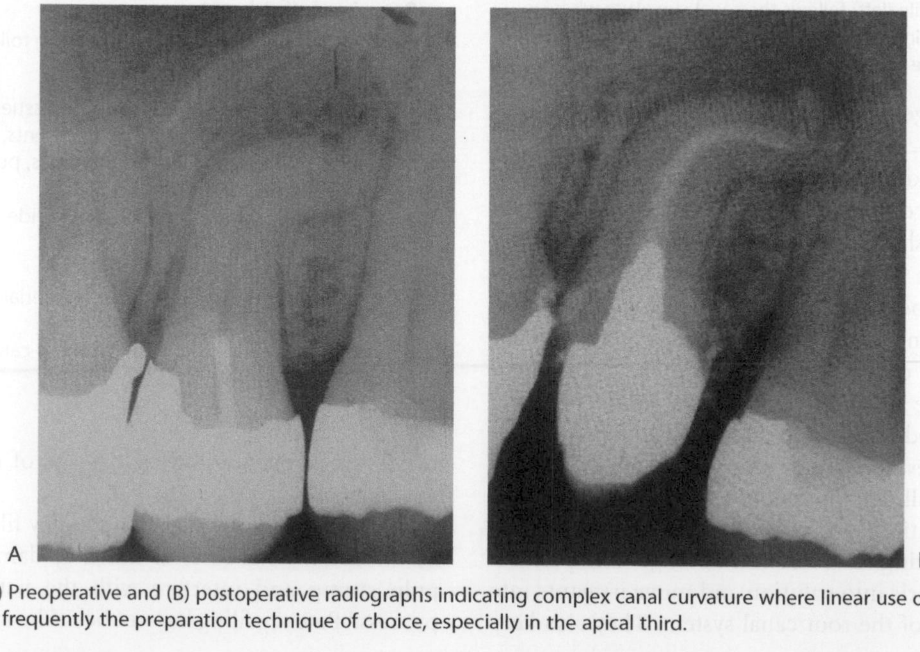

Figure 5.3 (A) Preoperative and (B) postoperative radiographs indicating complex canal curvature where linear use of hand instruments is frequently the preparation technique of choice, especially in the apical third.

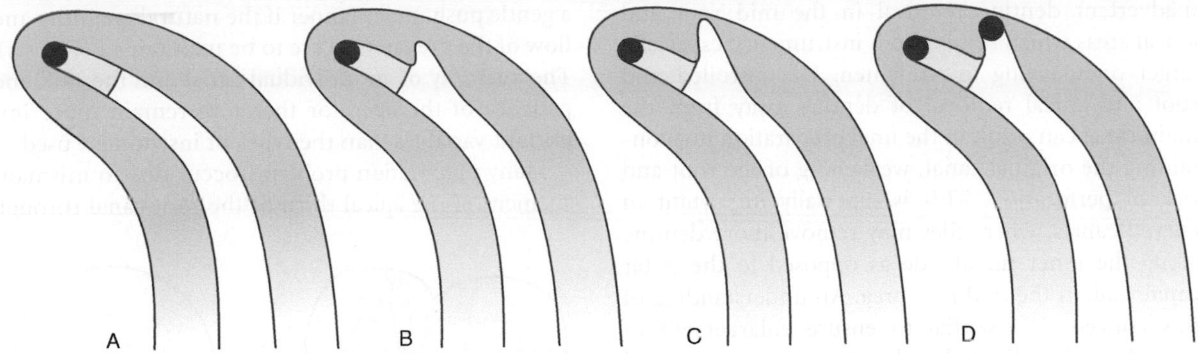

Figure 5.4 Examples of (A) blocked, (B) ledged, (C) internally transported and (D) perforated canal preparations.

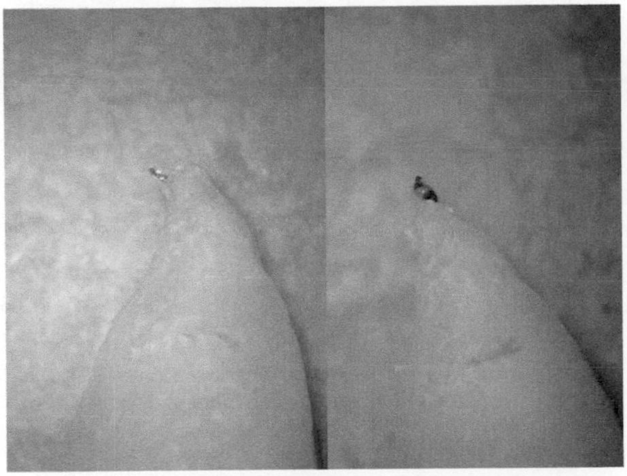

Figure 5.5 Correct (left) and incorrect (right) use of a patency file. The size 10 file (left) follows the canal curvature whereas the size 30 file (right) has ripped the apical foramen straightening the apical part of the canal, see Fig 5.6.

blockage, ledge formation, transportation or perforation (Fig. 5.4). Apical blockage frequently occurs as a result of packing dentine chips ahead of root canal instruments, especially in fine canals, and makes cleaning and shaping more difficult to achieve. Instruments used in an attempt to break up this debris may straighten or be deflected to the outer wall of the canal, thereby creating a ledge. Their further forceful use may subsequently create a perforation. These problems become more common as canal curvature increases but may be reduced by the careful use of a patency file (Fig. 5.5). These small (08, 10) precurved files are used in a push–pull motion in the long axis of the canal, with no rotation. Such files will prevent blockage, thereby reducing the incidence of ledges and perforations, stir debris into solution and move irrigants into deeper parts of the root canal system. They also keep the foramen open, allowing passage of exudate into the canal (Box 5.3).

Box 5.3 Patency filing

A patency file is a small file (08, 10) passed just out of the foramen using a push–pull action in the long axis of the canal.

Perceived advantages

The careful use of a patency file may give the following advantages:

- Preventing blockage
- Reducing the incidence of ledges or perforation
- Bringing debris into solution
- Helping to move irrigating solution deeper into the root canal system
- Keeping the foramen open, allowing exudates to pass into the canal.

Perceived disadvantages

Overuse of a patency file may create the following problems:[12]

- Direct physical trauma to the apical tissues
- Transportation of necrotic canal contents, dead or living organisms into the apical tissues, possibly resulting in persistent infection
- Bleeding into the root canal may provide nutrients for intracanal bacteria
- The foramen may be increased in size
- Increased risk of extruding filling material and irrigating solutions
- Creation of an oval foramen in curved canals may lead to a poor seal.

It has been suggested that a patency file should not be utilized in vital cases as this may damage the vital pulp stump and interfere with the natural healing process.[1] Patency filing has not been shown to increase

postoperative symptoms, although it may have the potential to extrude infected debris, albeit in small amounts, provided a crown-down instrumentation technique with copious irrigation has been employed. This technique, however, requires careful attention to detail as over-instrumentation with large instruments through the foramen will damage apical anatomy, produce mechanical irritation, periapical inflammation and, in infected cases, extrusion of infected debris. Other adverse effects resulting from apical over-instrumentation include overextension of filling points resulting in compression of the periradicular tissues, and chemical irritation from the extrusion of irrigating solutions, intracanal medicaments and root canal sealers beyond the apical foramen.

Root canal foramina are frequently not regular, and passing files through is unlikely to make them round, especially in the case of curved canals where the use of large files may cause tearing of the foramen by ripping it into an oval or tear-drop shape which is difficult to seal (Fig. 5.6). Foramen size has a natural variation which is increased in cases of incomplete root formation, the presence of apical periodontitis (which results in apical root resorption) or following apical surgery. There is no advantage in needlessly enlarging the foramen as this may irritate the supporting periodontal tissues, increase the likelihood of irrigant extrusion and make it difficult to ensure a continuously tapering preparation and apical seal. However, in infected cases, there may be advantages in removing bacteria and infected debris from the most apical part of the canal as remaining bacteria could act as a nidus of infection and jeopardize the outcome of treatment.

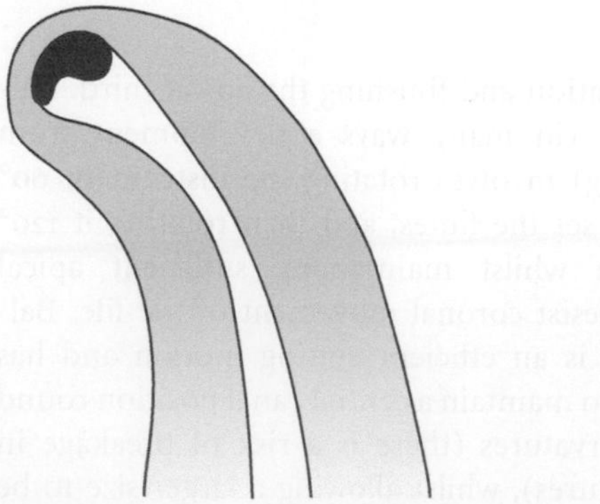

Figure 5.6 Tearing/ripping/zipping (external transportation) of the apical foramen which results in a tear-drop shape.

ARMAMENTARIUM FOR CLEANING AND SHAPING

Root canal instruments can be broadly categorized as those used by hand and those placed in a handpiece. Made from either stainless steel or nickel titanium, there are many different designs available. No attempt will be made to cover them all, rather some key features will be identified and explained.

Hand instruments

Hand instruments come in a variety of shapes and sizes, from barbed broaches, which are used to remove pulp tissue from large canals, to files and reamers. Most hand instruments are manufactured out of stainless steel (Fig. 5.7) with the most notable exceptions being hand GT (Greater Taper) and ProTaper files (Fig. 5.8). Hand stainless steel instruments have a taper of 0.02 mm per mm, are therefore quite parallel and are used successively shorter in the canal in a step-back manner to produce a continuously tapering preparation. When severe curvatures are present, nickel titanium 0.02 taper hand files (NitiFlex) may be used if desired, although small stainless steel hand files, used purely in a push–pull filing motion, are considered by many to be the preferred option. Much emphasis has

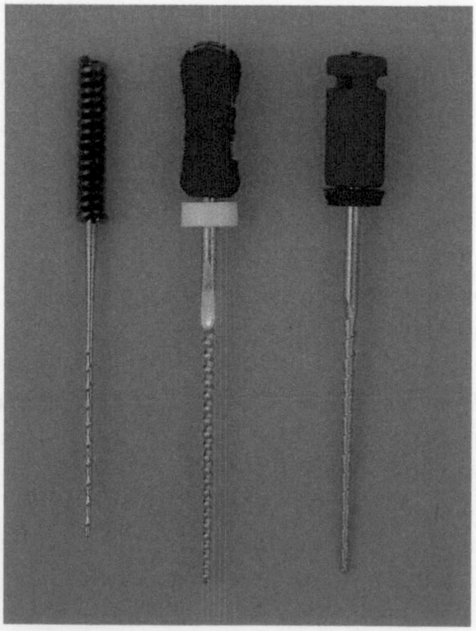

Figure 5.7 Examples of stainless steel hand instruments: barbed broach, K file, H file.

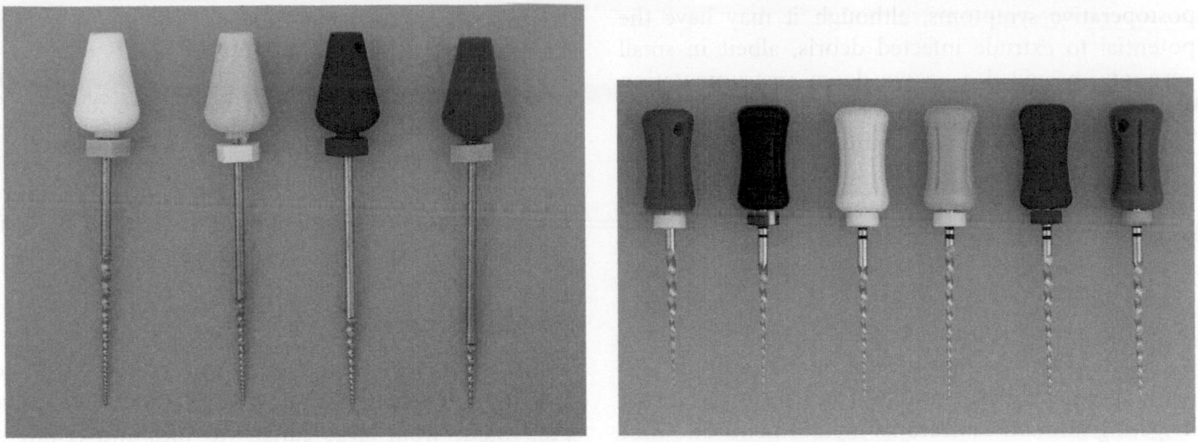
A B

Figure 5.8 Examples of nickel titanium hand files: (A) GT and (B) ProTaper.

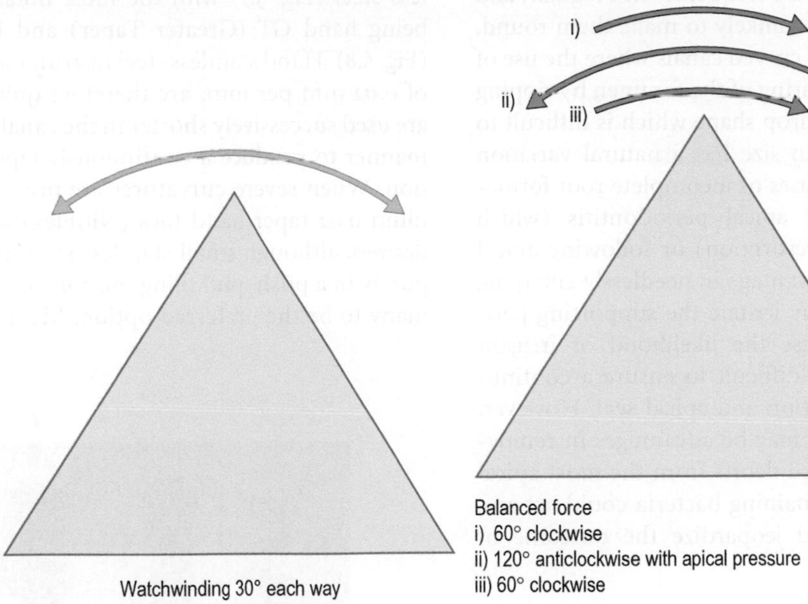

Figure 5.9 (A) Watchwinding and (B) balanced force hand file techniques.

been placed on instruments having safe tips to avoid gouging of canal walls. An important point, however, is that instruments can only gouge if they are forced into canals by dentists. When emphasis is placed on creating space laterally in the body of the canal prior to apical file advancement, problems are greatly reduced in this regard.

Hand files may be rotated, with the two most commonly used motions being watchwinding and balanced force (Fig. 5.9). Watchwinding refers to the gentle rotation of a file (30° each way). This motion is useful for all stages of canal preparation, especially initial negotiation and finishing the apical third. Balanced forces (in many ways a development from watchwinding) involves rotating the instrument 60° clockwise to set the flutes, and then rotating it 120° anticlockwise whilst maintaining sufficient apical pressure to resist coronal movement of the file. Balanced forces is an efficient cutting motion and has been shown to maintain a central canal position round moderate curvatures (there is a risk of breakage in severe curvatures), whilst allowing a larger size to be used apically (compared to other hand instrumentation techniques).

Table 5.1 Manufacturer's suggested criteria for use of GT files

Colour	Taper (mm/mm)	Use
White	0.06	Fine curved canals
Yellow	0.08	Lower anteriors, multirooted premolars, mesial roots of lower molars and buccal roots of upper molars
Red	0.10	Palatal roots of upper molars and distal roots of lower molars, single canal premolars, lower canines and upper anteriors
Blue	0.12	Big canals

Hand GT files are manufactured from nickel titanium which is noted for its hyperelasticity and shape memory. This increased flexibility has allowed files of a taper greater than the standard 0.02 mm per mm used for stainless steel instruments. Such greater tapered files range from 0.02 to 0.12 mm per mm taper. Hand GT files are available in a set of four, have a tip size of 20 and each file has a different taper: 0.06, 0.08, 0.10 and 0.12 mm/mm (see Fig. 5.8A). The files all have a maximum flute diameter of 1 mm to restrict coronal enlargement. The 20/06 has three times the rate of taper of a standard ISO 0.02 mm/mm taper file, the 20/08 has a taper of four times the standard, etc. The flutes of the files are machined in a reverse direction and so a reverse balanced force movement is recommended for their use, in view of the flute direction. The handle on these files has been increased in size in order to make this reverse balanced force manipulation easier. The manufacturer's suggested criteria for use of GT files is shown in Table 5.1 and the reverse balanced force (in view of the reverse flute pattern) method of use in Box 5.4.

Hand ProTapers are manufactured out of nickel titanium and have variable tapers ranging from 2 to 19% depending on the instrument in question. The three Shaper files (Sx, S1 and S2) have a profile similar to that of the Eiffel Tower and are used to prepare the coronal and middle thirds of the canal. The tips of these instruments should fit passively in the canal following a pathway previously established with stainless steel files. There are three Finisher files with the following tapers in their apical 3 mm: F1, 20/07; F2, 25/08; F3, 30/09; the files have a reverse taper decreasing to 0.55 mm/mm. The protocol for hand ProTaper use is outlined in Box 5.5. The files are used in a continuous rotation or half-turn watchwinding motion, taking care to ensure that the tip of the Shaper files does not bind.

Box 5.4 Reverse balance force method of manipulation of GT files

1. The apical size should be increased to at least 20 (preferably 25–30) to ensure the GT file tip is inactive and acts as a pilot. Straight line access should be assured.
2. Insert GT file until resistance to apical placement is met.
3. Rotate GT file in a counterclockwise direction to engage its flutes into dentine.
4. Rotate GT file in a clockwise direction, applying sufficient apical force to resist it backing out of canal.
5. Repeat above sequence until progress into canal stops.
6. Rotate in counterclockwise direction on removal, to load flutes and remove debris.
7. Check the apical 2 mm of the GT file frequently to ensure the flutes are free of debris and therefore not binding.
8. Clean the flutes, irrigate the canal and continue the counterclockwise/clockwise rotation.
9. Gauging and tuning completes GT file preparation, as not all foramina are size 20.

Box 5.5 Protocol for hand ProTaper use

1. Establish glide path in coronal two-thirds of canal with size 15 ISO hand file.
2. Use Gates-Gliddens to create straight line access where necessary and further enlarge coronal two-thirds.
3. Use S1 to length of 20 or 1 mm shorter 15 K file length.
4. Determine working length.
5. Confirm smooth glide path with 15/20 K file to working length.
6. Use S1 and S2 in that order to working length.
7. Re-check working length, use F1 to working length.
8. Step back F2 and F3 in 1 mm increments as required.
9. Thoroughly irrigate throughout.
10. Confirm apical shape with hand files 0.02 mm/mm taper.

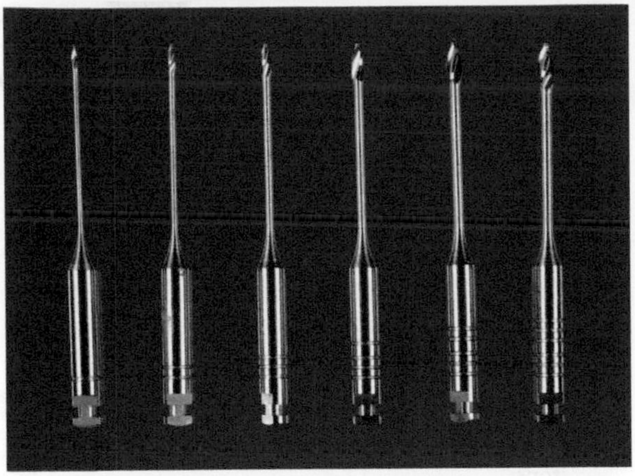

Figure 5.10 Range of Gates-Glidden burs, sizes 1–6.

Engine-driven instruments

Traditional engine-driven instruments include Gates-Glidden burs which have a flame-shaped head and a long thin shank, designed to fracture at the handpiece end. They are available in a range of sizes/numbers (Fig. 5.10) and may be used to relocate a canal away from the danger zone. However, care should be taken to avoid unnecessary over-enlargement.

In many ways rotary nickel titanium instruments have replaced Gates-Gliddens; however, these instruments still have a key role to play in access cavity refinement and preparation of the coronal one-third to two-thirds of the root canal. The recently introduced LAxxess burs (Fig. 5.11) have also been developed as a Gates-Glidden alternative to blend the coronal third of the root canal preparation with the access cavity and establish straight line access.

Problems of excessive dentine removal may be encountered with Gates-Gliddens, if they are used by dentists at too high a rotational speed. It is recommended, therefore, that they are used in a speed-reducing handpiece at a speed of 750–1000 rpm, brushing away from the danger areas of the canal, i.e. mesiobuccally in mesiobuccal canals, mesiolingually in mesiolingual canals, etc. (Fig. 5.12). Gates-Glidden Nos 6 and 5 should be used only on the walls of the access cavity, and No. 4 no deeper than the canal orifice. The No. 3 may be used a bud length deeper and the No. 2 may be taken to mid root, or near full length, in a straight canal. The No. 1 is quite fragile, but may be used at ultraslow speeds, provided it is loose in the

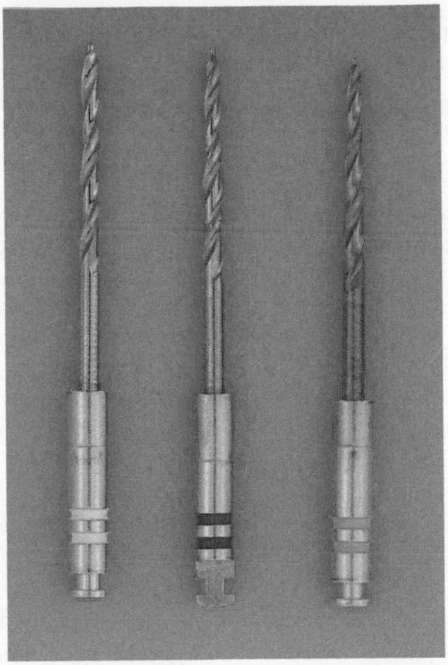

Figure 5.11 LAxxess burs.

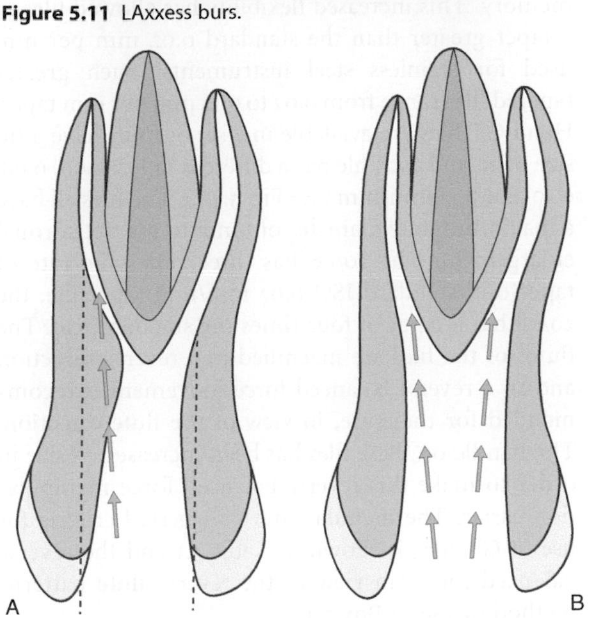

Figure 5.12 Upper molar tooth (A) before and (B) after removing overhanging triangles of dentine to improve straight line access.

canal. The most frequently used Gates-Gliddens are sizes 2, 3 and 4.

Rotary nickel titanium instruments

Nickel titanium (NiTi) has allowed the production of files that can be rotated continuously in a handpiece

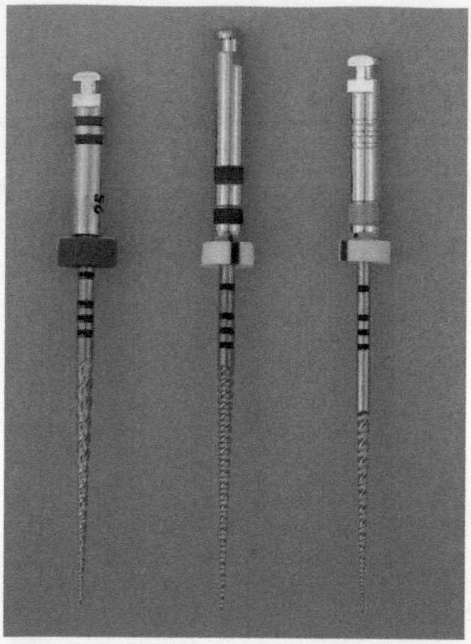

Figure 5.13 Range of single taper rotary NiTi instruments: K3 25/06, ProFile 25/06, GT 20/06.

through 360°. The advantages of the design of the present generation of rotary nickel titanium instruments include:

- increased debris removal, because of the continuous rotation
- reduced canal transportation
- smoother, faster canal preparation with less operator fatigue.

Numerous file designs are available — too many to be inclusive and all with their claimed advantages. It is important to understand the main role of these instruments is to enlarge, not negotiate, canals, thereby creating space and assisting in the cleaning and shaping of root canals, rather than completing the entire procedure. The anatomy of individual roots remains the major factor influencing instrument choice in root canal preparation.

Nickel titanium file designs may be characterised by taper or blade type.

- Single taper; K3, ProFile, GT (Fig. 5.13), Triniti and Race
- Multiple taper; ProTaper (Fig. 5.14)
- Radial land blades (Fig. 5.15); ProFile, K3, GT
- Cutting blades; ProTaper, Triniti

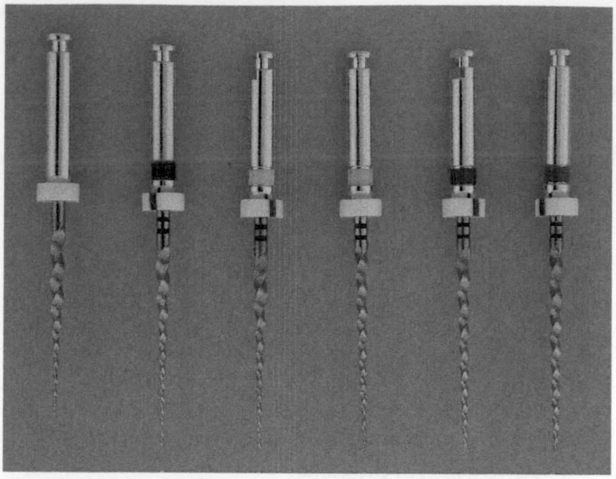

Figure 5.14 Range of ProTaper files which have a variable taper: three Shapers (Sx, S1, S2) and three Finishers (F1, F2, F3).

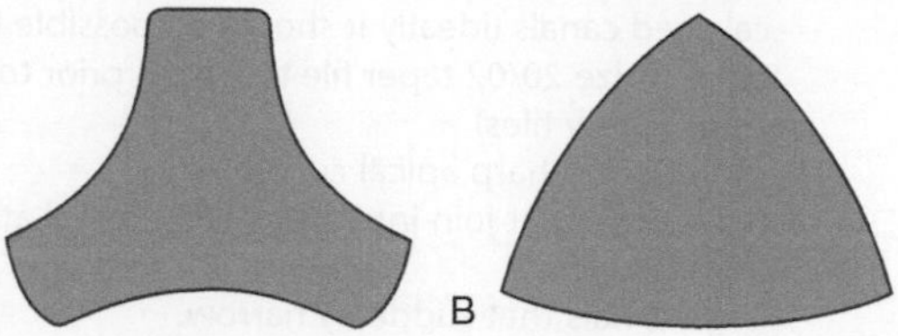

Figure 5.15 (A) ProFile radial lands and (B) ProTaper cutting edges.

Bladed instruments cut more efficiently but may inadvertently open the foramen if taken long repeatedly. Radial-landed instruments, although they cut more slowly, are safer in the apical region of the canal if working length is erroneously long, which can occur as progressive canal preparation straightens curved canals. There is a learning curve in the use of these instruments; once mastered, however, they are a quick, safe, effective, predictable and highly efficient way to prepare a root canal. However, the anatomy of an individual canal is a more important variable than the particular type of rotary NiTi instrument chosen as they all have limitations. Some special precautions for the use of automated NiTi instruments are outlined in Box 5.6.

Irrigation

Irrigating solutions are usually delivered using a syringe with a 27 or 28 gauge side-vented needle (Fig. 5.16). Care should be taken to ensure that the needle

Box 5.6 Precautions in the use of rotary NiTi instruments

1. Practise on extracted teeth first.
2. Ensure straight line access is present.
3. Use for canal enlargement, not negotiation. A NiTi file should never be taken where a hand file has not created a glide path.
4. Speed should be limited to 150–300 rpm in an electric handpiece.
5. Instruments must be used with a light touch, such as would not break a narrow lead propelling pencil.
6. A touch/retract, touch/retract technique is recommended; never keep an instrument at the same depth in the canal.
7. Advance files at no more than 1 mm at a time.
8. Limit the use of each file to approximately 4 seconds.
9. Damaged files should always be discarded.
10. It is important to be cautious in certain situations:
    — calcified canals (ideally it should be possible to place a size 20/02 taper file to length prior to using rotary files)
    — canals with sharp apical curvature
    — two canals that join into one smaller canal at a sharp angle
    — large canals that suddenly narrow.
11. Use files in a crown-down technique; large size to small size or more tapered to less tapered.
12. Clean files regularly and discard if damaged (bent or unwound). Do not overuse files (5–10 canals only).
13. Consider files as disposable instruments and factor this into the fee. Consider single patient use.
14. If in doubt, use hand instruments.

does not bind in the canal and that irrigating solution does not pass into periapical tissues causing a sodium hypochlorite (NaOCl) accident. The role of the irrigant is to flush out debris and provide lubrication for instruments. Specifically, an irrigant such as NaOCl will dissolve organic remnants and most importantly also has an antibacterial action. This may be used in a range of concentrations from 0.5 to 5.25%, 2.5% being the most popular. It is important that the irrigant is changed frequently; ideally irrigation should be performed between each file.

Ethylenediaminetetraacetic acid (EDTA) may be used to remove the smear layer, and alternating NaOCl with EDTA is a popular irrigation regime.

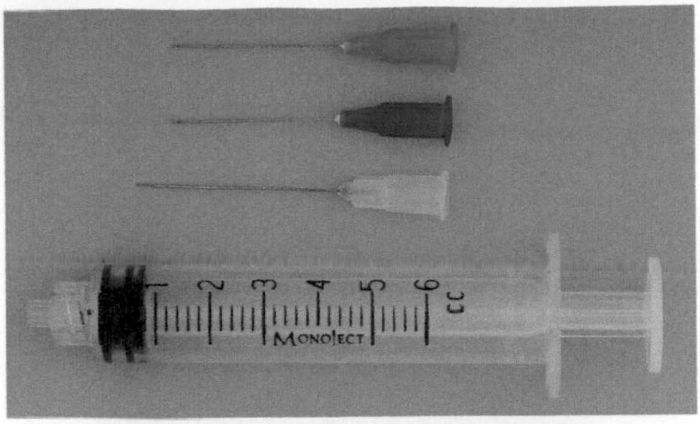

A

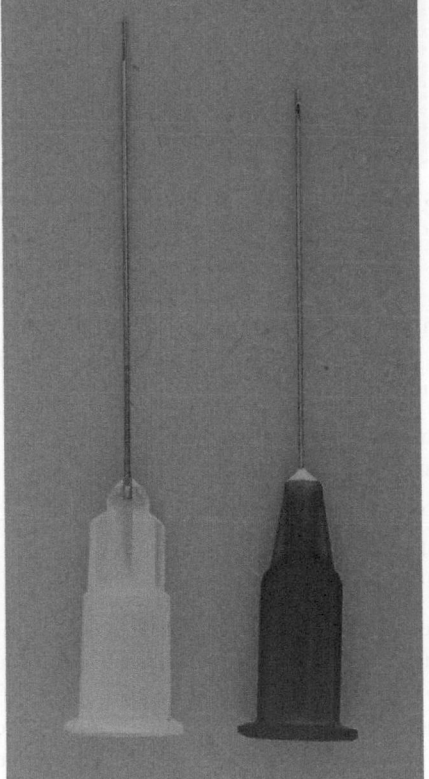
B

Figure 5.16 (A) Monoject irrigating syringe and endodontic irrigating needles. (B) Close-up of side-vented and maxi probe needle tips.

Other irrigating solutions include chlorhexidine, iodine potassium iodide (IKI) and mixture tetracycline acid and detergent (MTAD), with chlorhexidine being the most popular, especially in cases with open apices where it is felt there may be potential for extruding NaOCl into the periapical tissues. Chlorhexidine is beneficial in such situations as it is antibacterial when

used in similar concentrations to NaOCl without being caustic. It does not, however, have the same tissue-dissolving capabilities as NaOCl.

IKI (2–5%) may be used in therapy-resistant cases as it is effective against a broader range of bacteria. However, since it is dark brown in colour, it is advisable to rinse out thoroughly with NaOCl following its use. A further disadvantage of IKI is its allergenic potential and for this reason many operators prefer not to use it. MTAD is a new irrigation solution, advocated for a final rinse, and contains an acid to remove the smear layer and tetracycline to kill bacteria.

A most effective way of delivering irrigating solutions is through an ultrasonic handpiece (Fig. 5.17). Ultrasonic acoustic microstreaming has been shown to be effective at removing debris from canals provided the file is not constrained.[13,14] Care must be taken not to instrument the canal walls as this may cause irregularities or, in extreme cases of overuse, perforation. For this reason some operators prefer to use a plain nickel titanium finger spreader in the ultrasonic file holder.

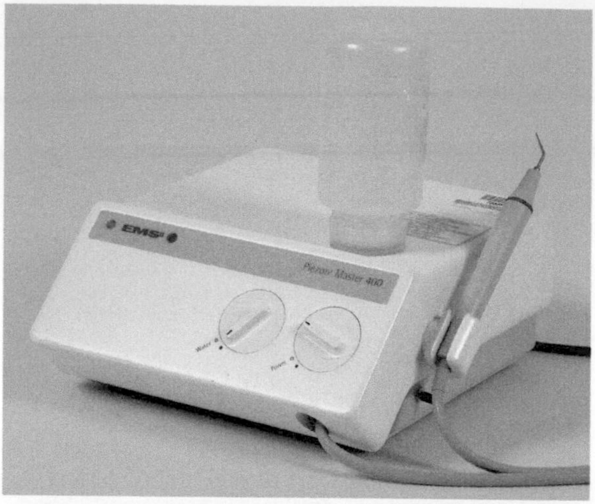

Figure 5.17 The Piezon Master 400 ultrasonic device. Such instruments create acoustic microstreaming within the irrigating solution, thereby enhancing cleaning.

REFERENCES

1. Bergenholtz G, Spanberg L. Controversies in endodontics. Crit Rev Oral Biol Med 2004; 15: 99–114.
2. Kuttler Y. Microscopic investigation of root apexes. J Am Dent Assoc 1955; 50: 544–552.
3. Dummer PMH, McGinn JH, Rees DG. The position and topography of the apical canal constriction and apical foramen. Int Endod J 1984; 17: 192–198.
4. Sjogren U, Hagglund B, Sundqvist G, Wing K. Factors affecting the long-term results of endodontic treatment. J Endod 1990; 16: 498–504.
5. Engstrom B, Spanberg L. Wound healing after partial pulpectomy. A histological study performed on contralateral tooth pairs. Odontol Tidskr 1967; 75: 5–18.
6. Nair PNR. Light and electron microscope studies of root canal flora and periapical lesions. J Endod 1987; 13: 29–39.
7. Nair PNR, Sjogren U, Kahnberg KE, Sundqvist G. Intraradicular bacteria and fungi in root-filled asymptomatic human teeth with therapy-resistant periapical lesions; a long-term light and electron microscopic follow-up study. J Endod 1990; 16: 580–588.
8. Hoskinson SE, Ng YL, Hoskinson AE, Moles DR, Gulabivala K. A retrospective comparison of outcome of root canal treatment using two different protocols. Oral Surg Oral Med Oral Pathol Oral Radiol Endod 2002; 93: 705–715.
9. Chugal NM, Clive JM, Spanberg LSW. Endodontic infection: some biologic and treatment factors associated with outcome. Oral Surg Oral Med Oral Pathol Oral Radiol Endod 2003; 96: 81–90.
10. Schilder H. Cleaning and shaping the root canal. Dent Clin North Am 1974; 18: 269–296.
11. Siquera JF, Barnett F. Interappointment pain: mechanisms, diagnosis, and treatment, Endod Topics 2004; 7: 93–109.
12. Haapasaalo M, Udnaes T, Endal U. Persistent, recurrent, and acquired infection of the root canal system post-treatment. Endod Topics 2003; 6: 29–56.
13. Lumley PJ, Walmsley AD, Walton RE, Rippin JW. Effect of precurving endosonic files on the amount of debris and smear layer remaining in curved root canals. J Endod 1993; 18: 616–619.
14. Lumley PJ, Walmsley AD, Walton RE, Rippin JW. Cleaning of oval canals using ultrasonic or sonic instrumentation. J Endod 1993; 19: 453–457.

6 Cleaning and shaping techniques

The underlying principles of cleaning, debridement and disinfection dictate that one is managing a microbial problem, and that antisepsis is a fundamental principle of root canal treatment. Teeth should be isolated with rubber dam to prevent contamination by saliva, and adequately restored to contain any surplus antibacterial irrigating solution (Fig. 6.1). A further important concept is that pulpal irritation may result in tertiary dentine deposition in the coronal part of the canal, restricting access to the apical third (Fig. 6.2) which represents the most important part of preparation. Thus coronal preparation may be considered as a means of gaining access to the apical infection. Some advantages of preparing canals coronal to apical are outlined in Box 6.1.

There are several methods of canal preparation and all have common objectives (Box 6.2). The sequence described here concentrates on coronal preparation, starting with exploration, initial coronal flaring, confirmation of straight line access, negotiation of the apical third, length refinement and completion of the preparation. It is recommended that straight line access and a patent canal are assured prior to the use of nickel titanium (NiTi) rotary instruments in the apical third of the canal as these steps significantly reduce the stress placed on instruments.

EXPLORATION AND INITIAL CORONAL FLARING

Root canals are infinitely variable in their shapes and sizes. Larger canals allow easy placement of instruments and irrigating solutions, whereas smaller ones require some initial coronal flaring prior to further canal exploration. Typically, stainless steel files (sizes 10, 15, 20 and 25) are used in the exploration phase of preparation, which aims to determine the width of the coronal one-third to two-thirds of the canal and to establish whether the file handles lie perpendicular to the occlusal surface of the tooth, indicating straight line access (SLA) is present. Care should be taken not to force instruments as this may result in a ledge, blockage, perforation or broken file, and a lubricating agent such as Glyde (Fig. 6.3) or RC Prep is recommended initially in constricted canals too narrow to receive an irrigating needle.

Should exploratory files pass freely down the canal, and SLA be confirmed, then more efficient rotary instruments may be employed. If SLA is not present then Gates-Glidden burs Nos 4, 3 and 2 should be used to improve the radicular access and straighten the coronal one-third to two-thirds of the canal and the files tried in again to check for SLA (Fig. 6.4). Gates-Gliddens may be used small size to large size or large to small, the decision being related to canal cross-sectional area, canal diameter and personal preference. Care should be taken to establish whether the access cavity requires modification, particularly in the marginal ridge areas, to remove unnecessary pressure on rotary files. It is important that rotary NiTi files are not used prior to confirmation of SLA.

Tight resistance to file advancement indicates that the rate of taper of the instrument exceeds that of the canal. In such situations it is necessary to use larger stainless steel files, stepped back (typically 10–35) to free the initial negotiation file from binding coronally, and to make file advancement easier. In tight, more constricted canals, small files need to be used carefully, with a watchwinding action to open and flare the canal in its coronal aspects, cutting laterally before apical, and with particular attention being paid to more frequent recapitulation and irrigation. These small files should be stepped back gradually and not forced to predetermined lengths, i.e. instruments are being used in a step-back manner, but shape is being created crown-down. On occasion, it may be necessary to use stainless steel files sizes 06 and 08 to negotiate canals. Situations where this approach may be indicated include mesiobuccal (MB) Zs and very curved canals. After initial coronal flaring, smaller files will pass

Box 6.1 Advantages of pre-enlargement and establishment of straight line access

Biological

1. Pulp tissue, bacteria and related irritants in the coronal area of the canal are removed early in the procedure.
2. Space is created for an increased volume of irrigating solution, which can be effective deeper in the canal system.
3. Files pass through irrigant solution before advancing into the apical third.
4. The increased space allows files to fit passively in the canal, allowing debris to pass coronally, thus reducing extrusion of infected material into the periapical tissues.

Mechanical

5. Coronal binding of file flutes is decreased, thereby increasing tactile sense and control when using files in the apical third.
6. A more direct path to the canal terminus is established prior to establishing working length, which leads to greater accuracy in the preparation of curved canals.
7. Precurved files are easier to insert, remain curved and are therefore more effective in apical canal exploration.

Box 6.2 Objectives of canal preparation

- To remove infected tissue from the root canal
- To create space, thereby facilitating the use and effectiveness of irrigating solutions
- To create space for the placement of intervisit intracanal medicaments
- To create a suitable shape to receive obturating materials

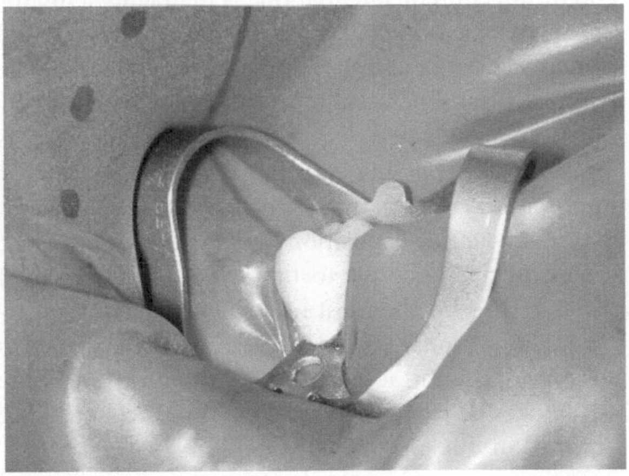

Figure 6.1 Rubber dam isolation is a key aspect of an aseptic technique.

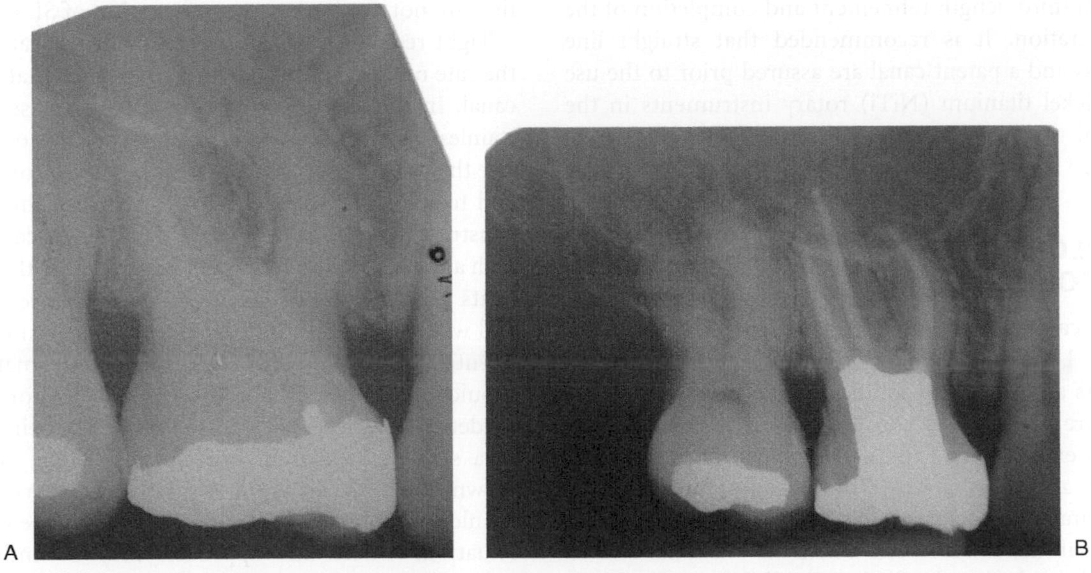

Figure 6.2 (A) Radiograph showing how pulpal irritation can lead to tertiary dentine deposition in the coronal part of the canal, making canal identification and negotiation more difficult. (B) Postoperative radiograph.

deeper down the canal. It may be necessary to repeat this sequence a few times before instruments can be taken to length.

NEGOTIATION OF THE APICAL THIRD, PATENCY AND WORKING LENGTH

Once some preparation has been performed coronally, then an 08 or 10 file can be advanced apically using lubricant as necessary to explore apical anatomy and see if any complexities exist. In a tooth with a large canal, or one where there is already plenty of shape/space, the file may pass straight to length. If, however, the file is loose in the canal but then hits against an obstruction, this usually indicates a sudden change in direction (curvature) of the canal or a division. In such circumstances the taper of the canal is greater than that of the file and it is necessary to curve the apical 1–2 mm of the file and make an attempt to pick and feel for the canal path. When it is found, a slight (starting at <1 mm) push–pull movement should be employed to smooth the path of the file. Careful evaluation of these exploratory files provides detailed information on apical canal anatomy, especially in regard to curvatures and divisions.

It is essential that care is taken over determination of canal length and it is understood that this can change, becoming shorter during preparation, especially in curved canals. Patency should be assured with an 08 or 10 ISO 0.02 taper stainless steel file and the provisional working length established with an apex locator (files larger than a size 10 should not be used through the foramen). Electronic apex locators have a lip hook and a clip or fork which contacts the file shaft (Fig. 6.5). As the file approaches the foramen the resistance or impedance changes and a visual display indicates file advancement. Apex locator displays vary and do not necessarily indicate the same file position relative to the apex; it is therefore important to be familiar with the nuances of the particular device being used. Care must be taken to ensure that the pulp chamber is dry and that there is minimal fluid in the root canals, as excess fluid may cause a false reading by creating a short circuit. This may be a particular problem in heavily restored or crowned teeth. It is

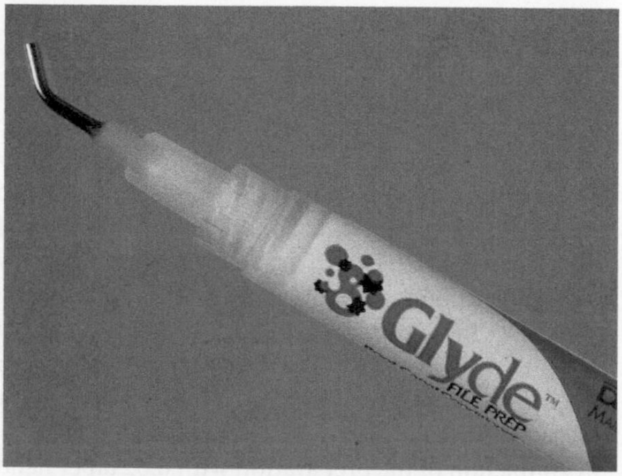

Figure 6.3 Popular lubricating agent, Glyde.

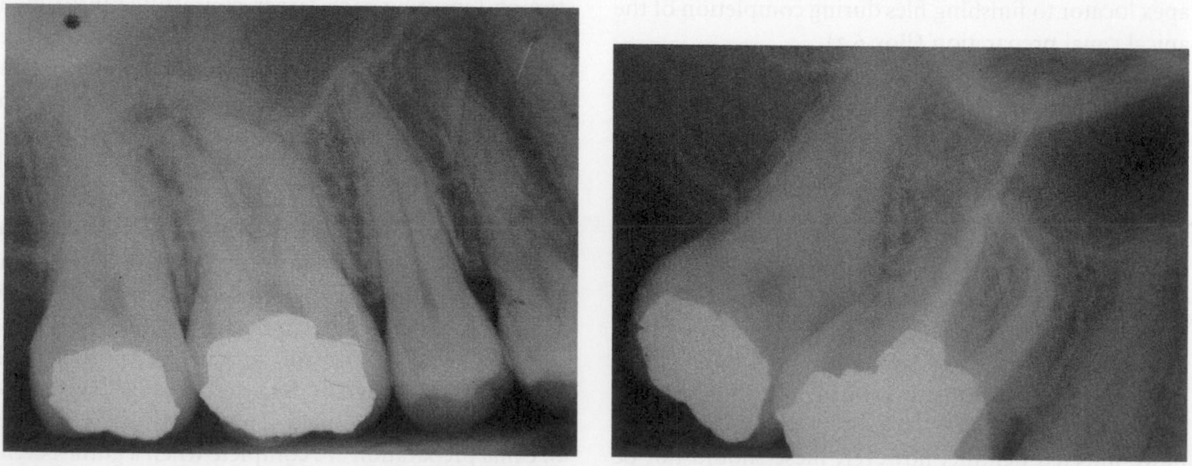

A

B

Figure 6.4 (A) Absence of and (B) presence of straight line access.

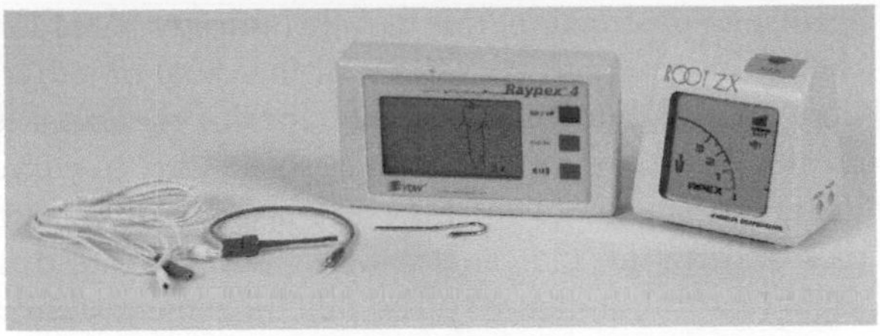

Figure 6.5 Two popular apex locators, the Raypex 4 and Root ZX. The lip clip is moistened and placed around the lower lip and the clip is attached to the metallic part of the root canal file.

Box 6.3 Use of electronic apex locators

- Ensure the floor of the pulp chamber is dry and there is minimal fluid in the root canals
- Avoid contact with metallic restorations
- File sizes closer to the foramen width normally give more consistent readings

usual to check the reproducibility of the reading with increasing file sizes (08, 10, 15 or 20, depending on canal size). A working length radiograph is still recommended, as this provides additional information — for example, an indication of direction and degree of curvature and information on possible unidentified canals. Apex locators allow greater accuracy in root canal preparation and provide the opportunity to monitor changes in canal length that may occur during the preparation of curved canals as they straighten. It is particularly advantageous to attach the apex locator to finishing files during completion of the apical canal preparation (Box 6.3).

COMPLETION OF THE CANAL PREPARATION

Stainless steel hand instruments

Much of the description so far has dealt with the use of stainless steel hand instruments to provide a platform for finishing the canal, either conventionally with hand instruments or using rotary NiTi instruments in a crown-down manner to perform the bulk of the canal preparation prior to hand file finishing. Larger apical preparation sizes have been shown to remove more infected dentine; however, these should not be beyond what is considered safe — for example, apical

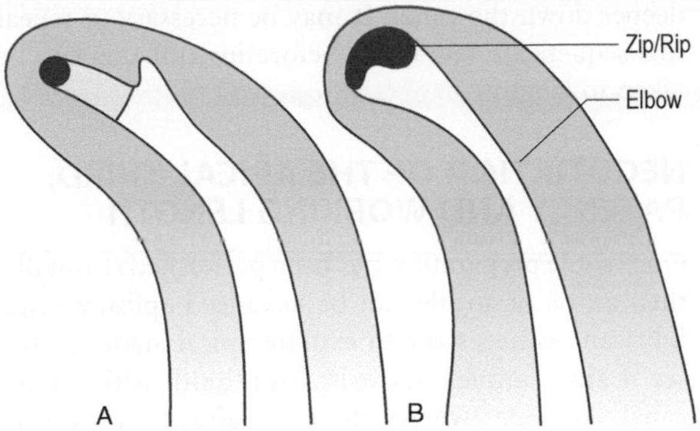

Figure 6.6 Common problems in the preparation of curved canals: (A) ledge; (B) hourglass shape showing elbow and externally transported foramen (zip/rip). This damage has occurred as the result of using increasingly larger files past the foramen.

preparation of curved canals is generally kept small, usually a size 30 or, in very curved canals, a size 25. The use of excessively large files in curved canals may produce internal transportation and a ledge or an hourglass shape, termed a zip and elbow (Fig. 6.6). If large files are taken long past the foramen then they will cause ripping of the foramen into a tear-drop shape. On the contrary, repeated use of a series of small files will result in a smooth canal preparation larger than the file used, which will be appropriate for the particular root.

Completion of the preparation with 0.02 taper hand instruments involves gauging (discovering how big the foramen is), determining the file that binds approximately 0.5 mm short of the full canal length and then tuning (ensuring each larger consecutive instrument uniformly backs out of the canal).[1] ISO stainless steel or NiTi 0.02 taper files (20–60) are used with a light touch until the instruments step back in 0.5–1 mm increments, or 0.25 mm increments for the apical area, to create additional resistance form in canals with large foramina, such as those with incomplete root development, apical resorption or surgically altered apices. It may be necessary to recapitulate, i.e. reintroduce the previously placed series of instruments to further refine the preparation until files sit at the desired level and blend apical preparation with the coronal. Finally, the foramen is gauged again and the apical 2–3 mm refined. The mechanical objectives of canal preparation are complete when a gutta-percha cone can be fitted, and the biological objectives are

satisfied when the canal has been optimally cleaned with the majority of bacteria eliminated.

An alternative hand-finishing technique is to use hand GT files to simplify step back and blend the apical and middle thirds of the canal preparation, as described previously. It is important that some apical preparation has been performed, preferably to a size 25 or 30, before GT files are used, as this ensures the tips are not engaged. GTs may be used large taper to small, or small to large depending on personal preference, taking care to ensure finishing is completed with 0.02 taper files to gauge the foramen and ensure apical taper/resistance form. Hand ProTaper files could also be used.

Rotary nickel titanium instruments

Technique for the use of rotary nickel titanium (NiTi) instruments is evolving continuously as greater understanding is gained of how best to use them safely. However, it is clear that canal anatomy, especially oval canals and hidden curvatures, is a major factor in file performance, hence the importance of thorough exploration with hand files prior to using these instruments. A quality electric motor (Fig. 6.7) with speed reduction handpiece with high torque is recommended for use with NiTi instruments to allow appropriate speeds (150–300 rpm) to be used. Pre-enlargement, coronal flaring, establishment of SLA and a crown-down approach are now recognized as being important considerations in getting best results and limiting instrument failure, all of which have been described previously. Rotary NiTi files should not be used to negotiate canals as they need to follow a pathway. A rotary file must never be taken where a hand file has not been; the creation of a pathway or glide path (minimum size 15, preferably 20) for the instruments to follow is essential as these instruments are for canal enlargement, not canal negotiation.

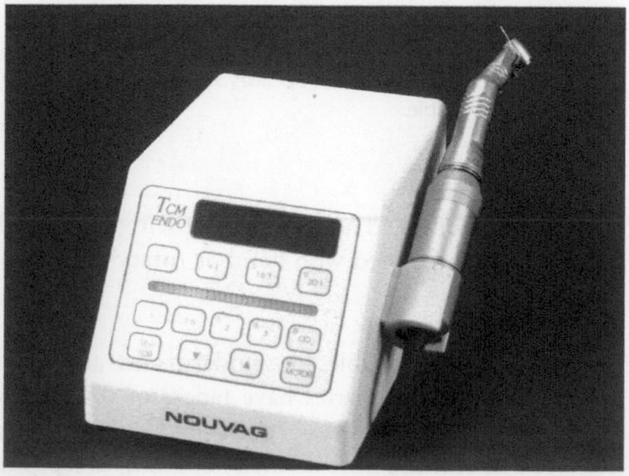

Figure 6.7 Electric endodontic motor, the Nouvag.

Instruments must be used with a light touch, similar to that which would be used with a narrow lead propelling pencil. Introduction into the canal should be gradual, using a touch/retract motion no more than 1 mm at a time. The instrument should be continuously introduced and removed, never being held at the same point in the canal. Their use should be preceded by irrigation and followed by a small hand instrument to move irrigating solutions deeper into the canal system and maintain canal patency.

Nickel titanium has good shape memory, which makes it difficult to see when files are fatigued. Canal length, curvature and calcification all influence fatigue and thought should be given to considering NiTi instruments, indeed all instruments, as single patient use. Instruments that show any sign of damage should be discarded, as should ones used in highly calcified or severely curved canals.

Preparation is not completed once the first rotary gets to length, and care should be taken to gauge and prepare the apical few millimetres of the canal by hand or further rotary instrumentation, as frequently the apical canal wall will not have been touched with the first rotary file. Hand finishing is indicated in cases of complex anatomy where a smooth glide path has been difficult to achieve due to canal branches or curvatures (Fig. 6.8).

Preparation techniques

Three techniques with which the authors are familiar and teach routinely will be outlined here: ProFile, rotary GTs and ProTaper. Prerequisites for all techniques are:

- straight line access
- a patent canal
- a glide path.

It is recommended, however, that such preparation techniques are best learned on hands-on courses and practised on extracted teeth prior to use on patients.

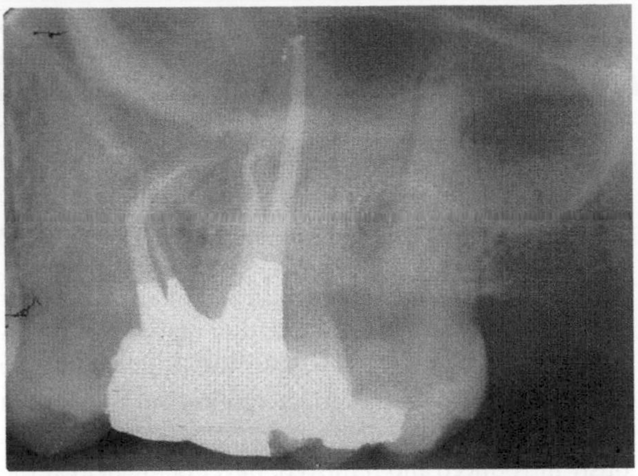

Figure 6.8 Example of complex anatomy where a combination of rotary NiTi and hand instruments is advised, especially in the distobuccal root.

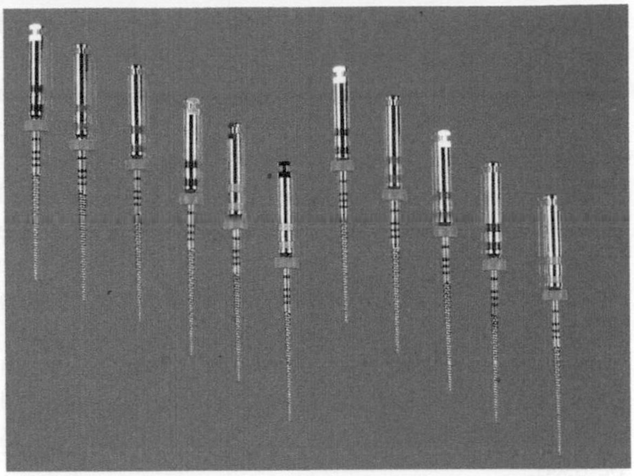

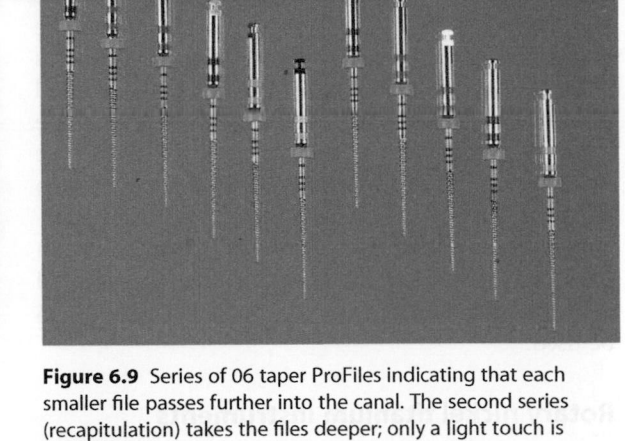

Figure 6.9 Series of 06 taper ProFiles indicating that each smaller file passes further into the canal. The second series (recapitulation) takes the files deeper; only a light touch is required.

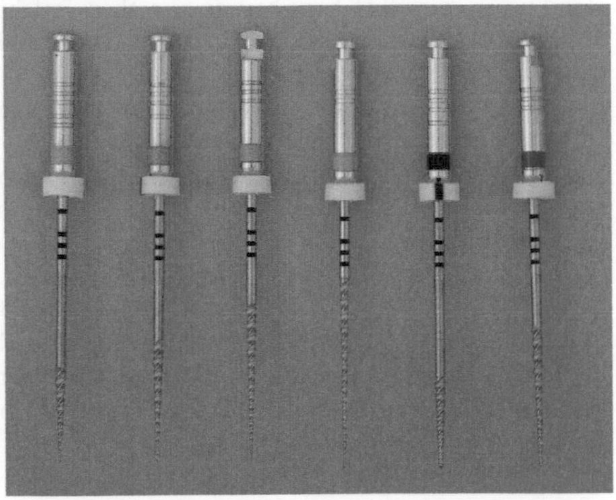

Figure 6.10 The Standard 20 GT series (tapers 0.10, 0.08, 0.06, 0.04) together with examples of increased tip sizes, 30/06 and 40/04. Accessory rotary GT files, tip sizes 35, 50, 70, all taper; 0.12 are also available.

Many operators prefer to have negotiated the canal fully to length with stainless steel files before using rotary NiTi instruments, thus ensuring a glide path has been created and straight line access confirmed (using gates or diamonds as appropriate). Practising in this conservative manner provides a thorough understanding of canal anatomy and reduces many of the problems that may be encountered with NiTi files.

ProFile

ProFile rotary NiTi instruments may be used in conjunction with Gates-Glidden burs or Orifice Shapers following the establishment of straight line access and a glide path. Preparation proceeds crown-down, using large instruments before small, with many operators preferring to use the 06 taper series (40, 35, 30, 25, 20, 15; Fig. 6.9) in view of the increased taper compared to the 04 files.[2] It has been suggested, however, that using files of one taper may increase the risk of fracture through taper lock (increased binding along the length of the file) and that alternating between 06 and 04 tapers may reduce this problem, as fewer file flutes are binding at any one time. Popular alternating taper series include Orifice Shapers 5 (60/08), 4 (50/07), 3 (40/06), 2 (30/06); ProFile 25/06, 25/04, 20/06, 20/04[3] in combination with GT files to produce deeper shape as required; or K3 series Orifice Openers 25/10, 25/08, K3, 35/04, 30/06, 25/04, 20/06, 20/04.[4] In all instances, further recapitulations of the file series may be required until a 20/06 or 25/06 goes to 0.5 mm short of apex locator length. The foramen is then gauged and preparation completed with hand or rotary files.

Rotary GT files

These files are available in standard and accessory series. The standard series have tapers of 0.10, 0.08, 0.06 and 0.04 with tip sizes of 20, 30 and 40 (Fig. 6.10); all have a maximum flute diameter of 1 mm, except the 40/10 which has a maximum flute diameter of 1.25 mm.

The accessory series have a taper of 0.12, and a tip size of 35, 50 or 70, with a maximum flute diameter of 1.5 mm. The accessory series are rarely used in view of their size and stiffness. It is recommended that the canal be negotiated to length with at least a size 15 file, and straight line access confirmed prior to introducing the rotary files. Preparation proceeds crown-down, using larger to smaller taper with the 20 series 0.10, 0.08, 0.06, 0.04, recapitulating through the series as necessary.[5] Once the appropriate taper rotary file is at length, the foramen is gauged and the preparation completed by hand or using the appropriate tip size GT of the same taper as the one that initially went to length.

ProTaper

ProTaper (Fig. 6.11) is a relatively new and innovative instrument design that has a variable taper along its length, no radial lands and cuts very effectively. There are three Shaper files and three Finisher files.[6] The method of use is different from ProFiles and GTs in that ProTaper Shaper files are taken to resistance and then brushed laterally, rather like Gates-Gliddens, away from furcal areas. Each ProTaper Shaper creates its own crown-down in view of the variable taper. Finishers are taken short of the Shapers, not brushed, and removed immediately they have reached length. The technique is outlined below.

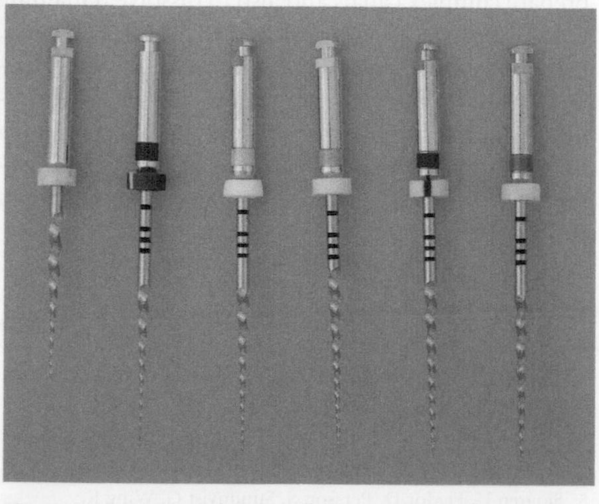

Figure 6.11 Series of ProTaper files: three Shapers (Sx, S1, S2) and three Finishers with apical 3 mm tapers, respectively, of F1 (20/07), F2 (25/08), F3 (30/09).

1. Explore the canals with stainless steel 10, 15 and 20 files; use Gates-Gliddens to refine the access if SLA is not present; establish a glide path.
2. The S1 is taken to the approximate glide path depth of the size 20 file, brushing laterally as resistance is met.
3. The S2 is taken to the same length as the S1; alternatively the Sx file may be used. The Sx should be placed carefully, lifted, and brushed laterally to relocate the canal. The Sx is not used first because this may cause the tip to bind and break, and is only taken deeper once the tip is free. The Sx is never taken into coronal curvature as the tip may break. Use gates instead to create straight line access. The Sx may be used later to create more shape. Do not overdo it, however, as removing dentine weakens the root, making it more susceptible to fracture.
4. Establish electronic apex locator (EAL) length.
5. Confirm glide path with 15 and 20, then take S1 and S2 to 0.5 mm short of EAL length, brushing as necessary. Do not brush at length, stop brushing 1 mm short.
6. Recheck EAL length as curved canals will be shorter following use of the Shaper files.
7. Take F1 to 0.5 mm short of refined EAL and remove immediately.
8. Take F2 to 1 mm short of F1, and F3 a further 1 mm short (i.e. step Finishers back at 1 mm intervals; they can always be taken deeper with care later if required). Never take Finishers to the same length as the Shapers, do not linger at length and do not brush. Alternatively, a hybrid technique may be employed using GT files or ProFiles to finish the rotary canal preparation.
9. Complete preparation by hand, gauge and tune.

Caution!

Much of this chapter has been based around mechanical aspects of canal instrumentation; however, there is a need for caution. Rotary NiTi files make canal preparation easier by providing a shape that easily accepts a filling point and looks aesthetic on a radiograph. The reality may, however, be different, as rotary files ream a round hole and debris is frequently pushed laterally into canal recesses (Fig. 6.12). This

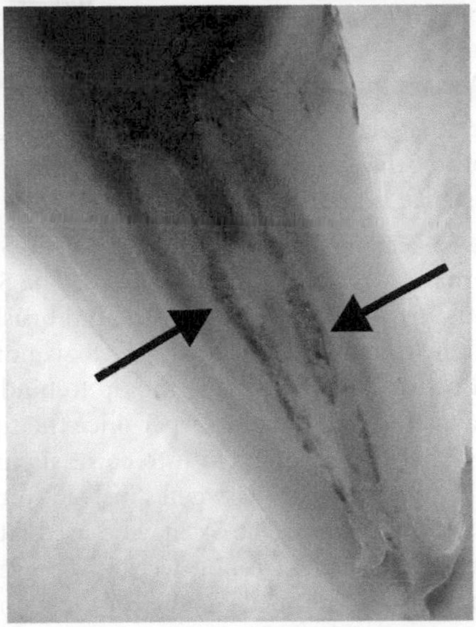

Figure 6.12 Cleared tooth following rotary preparation showing debris pushed laterally into recesses and untouched walls in oval canals.

debris should be removed using hand or ultrasonic instrumentation and copious irrigation and is another reason that rotary preparation should always be finished by hand, with particular attention being paid to oval recesses. As many rotary techniques reduce the time required to prepare the canal, it is therefore important to ensure that adequate active irrigation is performed once the intracanal space/shape has been created prior to intervisit dressing or obturation.

Single versus multiple visit treatment

Root canal therapy may be performed in one visit if time allows completion of cleaning and disinfection and the canals can be dried. However, it is important that procedures are not rushed and corners cut because completion of the treatment in one visit has become the objective, as opposed to thorough debridement, disinfection and obturation of the root canal system.

Several advantages exist in carrying out procedures over two visits, including the opportunity to:

- enhance root canal disinfection
- observe the progress of healing[7]
- check preparation
- search for additional canals.

Calcium hydroxide is the preferred intervisit medicament. This compound has a high pH and will further help to reduce the bacterial flora and dissolve tissue following instrumentation and irrigation, and is particularly indicated in cases of apical periodontitis. Care needs to be taken to ensure that a sound coronal seal of 3–4 mm in length is present to prevent recontamination of the canal between visits. It is also usual to place a small pledget of cotton wool, foam or gutta-percha prior to placing the interappointment temporary seal in order to prevent inadvertent dropping of material into the canal between visits, or during subsequent removal. A popular alternative favoured by many is to use Cavit G under the temporary seal for its improved sealing ability compared to cotton wool etc.

From the biological standpoint, the choice of single versus multiple visit therapy should be based on the disease process. Thus, in vital non-infected cases, treatment should be completed as soon as possible, preferably in one visit if time allows. In teeth with complex anatomy, $Ca(OH)_2$ may be placed because of the increased treatment time to identify, negotiate and prepare complex canals and also to dissolve remaining pulp or reduce bleeding. However, in infected cases, there are strong arguments for multiple visit treatment, with $Ca(OH)_2$ therapy to reduce bacterial infection, as instrumentation and NaOCl have been shown to not always eliminate intracanal bacteria, and infection at the time of obturation affects the outcome of treatment.[8]

REFERENCES

1. Ruddle CJ. Endodontic canal preparation, breakthrough cleaning and shaping strategies. Dent Today 1994; 20: 76–83.
2. Kavanagh D, Lumley PJ. An in-vitro evaluation of canal preparation using Profile .04 and .06 taper instruments. Endod Dent Traumatol 1998; 14: 16–20.
3. Hoskinson AE. Personal communication, 1998.
4. Barnett F. Personal communication, 2002.
5. Buchanan LS. The art of endodontics: files of greater taper. Dent Today 1996; 17: 74–81.
6. Ruddle CJ. The ProTaper technique. Endod Pract 2002; 5: 22–30.
7. Trope M, Bergenholtz G. Microbiological basis of endodontic treatment: can a maximal outcome be achieved in one visit? Endod Topics 2002; 1: 40–53.
8. Sjogren U, Figdor D, Persson S, Sundqvist G, Wing K. Influence of infection at the time of root filling on the outcome of endodontic treatment of teeth with apical periodontitis. Int Endod J 1997; 30: 297–306.

7 Root canal obturation

It is important to appreciate that despite optimal cleaning and shaping techniques some residual bacteria may remain in the root canal system. Generally, these bacteria do not cause clinical problems. The aims of canal obturation are summarized in Box 7.1.

The objective of canal obturation, therefore, is to incarcerate any remaining bacteria in an environment where they cannot thrive and provide a fluid-tight seal in the canal from the coronal to apical aspect. Although the apical seal is important, recent emphasis has been placed on the need for a coronal seal as contamination usually starts coronally, especially from saliva. If the coronal seal of the temporary or final restoration is poor, contamination of the root canal filling may occur, eventually leading to failure.

REQUIREMENTS BEFORE ROOT CANAL FILLING

The tooth must be asymptomatic, chemomechanical preparation complete and the root canal dry before a root filling is inserted. Any serous exudate from the periapical tissues indicates the presence of inflammation. If there is persistent seepage, calcium hydroxide may be used as a root canal dressing until the root canal is dry. It is advisable to recheck the canal length in situations of persistent seepage as this may frequently result from over-instrumentation and damage to the periapical tissues. If it is not possible to dry the canal, therapy-resistant or extraradicular infection may be present. Consideration should be given to further treatment, i.e. surgery or extraction. The criteria for obturation are summarized in Box 7.2 and the ideal properties of root canal filling materials and sealers in Boxes 7.3 and 7.4.

All sealers are irritant when first mixed, but this generally subsides.

TYPES OF ROOT FILLING MATERIAL

Root filling materials available can be summarized as follows:

- *Solid and semisolid materials* (e.g. gutta-percha and silver points; Figs 7.1 and 7.2). Silver points are not recommended as they do not seal the canal laterally or coronally and may cause tooth or gingival staining.
- *Sealers and cements* (e.g. Tubliseal, AH Plus, pulp canal sealer, Roth's sealer; Figs 7.3 and 7.4). Grossman's sealer and AH Plus have also been shown to be effective against *Enterococcus faecalis* in an in vitro study.[1] Recently, resin-based sealers have been introduced (Fig. 7.5), and whilst these are still comparatively new, a contemporary study has shown that they can be clinically adequate.[2]
- *Medicated pastes* (e.g. N2, Endomethosone, Spad, Kri). These are not recommended as they may contain paraformaldehyde which is cytotoxic.

GUTTA-PERCHA FILLING TECHNIQUES

Each of the techniques (except where indicated) will produce acceptable clinical results if used correctly. Following the introduction of increased taper files, numerous gutta-percha points have been produced to match the files. Proponents exist for the different techniques, although personal preference usually determines the final choice:

- Single cone (not recommended as it does not seal laterally and coronally)
- Lateral condensation
- Thermomechanical compaction
- Vertical condensation
- Thermoplasticized gutta-percha
- Carrier-based techniques
- Barrier techniques.

Preparation for obturation

The same principles of tooth isolation apply to the obturation phase as for preparation. It is vital that

Box 7.1 Obturation

Obturation has four aims:

— to prevent remaining bacteria and their toxins percolating into the periradicular tissues
— to seal remaining bacteria within the root canal system in an environment where they cannot thrive
— to prevent percolation of periradicular exudate, a nutrient source for remaining bacteria, into the root canal space[3]
— to prevent reinfection of the cleaned canal system from the coronal aspect.[4]

Box 7.2 Criteria to be met prior to obturation

- Tooth asymptomatic
- Temporary dressing intact
- No sinus
- Root canal dry

Box 7.3 Properties of an ideal root canal filling material

A root canal filling material should:

— be easily introduced into the root canal
— not irritate periradicular tissues
— be dimensionally stable
— seal the root canal laterally, apically and coronally
— be impervious to moisture
— be sterile or easily sterilized before insertion
— be bacteriostatic
— be radiopaque
— not stain tooth structure or gingival tissues
— be easily removed from the canal as necessary
— have a long shelf life
— adhere to dentine
— allow good length control.

Box 7.4 Properties of an ideal root canal sealer

An ideal sealer should:

— satisfy the requirements of a root filling material
— provide good adhesion to the canal wall
— have fine powder particles to allow easy mixing or be a two paste system
— have adequate working time
— expand whilst setting.

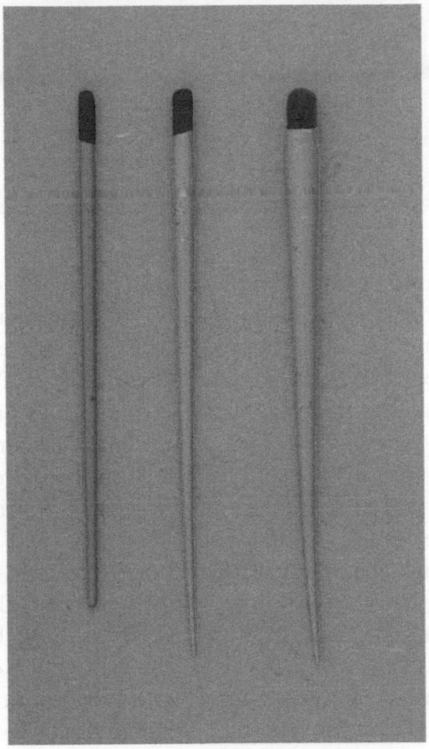

Figure 7.1 Gutta-percha points in standard 02 taper and greater taper: 04 and 06.

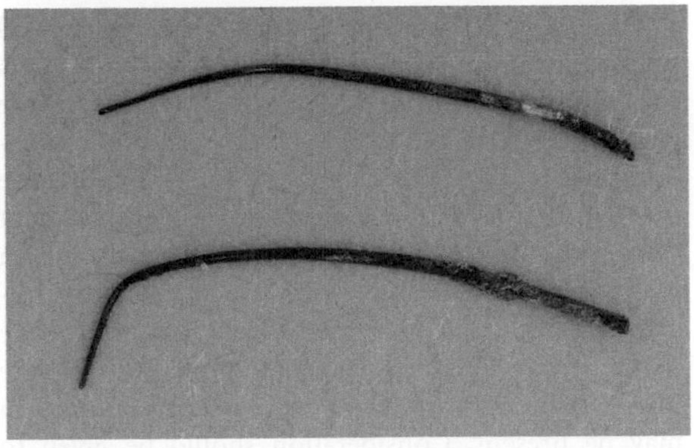

Figure 7.2 Failed silver points, note corrosion.

contamination of the root canal from saliva is prevented during this stage with rubber dam which will also contain irrigant solutions during final irrigation of the canals.

Lateral condensation of gutta-percha

This technique has been long established and has a good track record. It is often used as the standard to

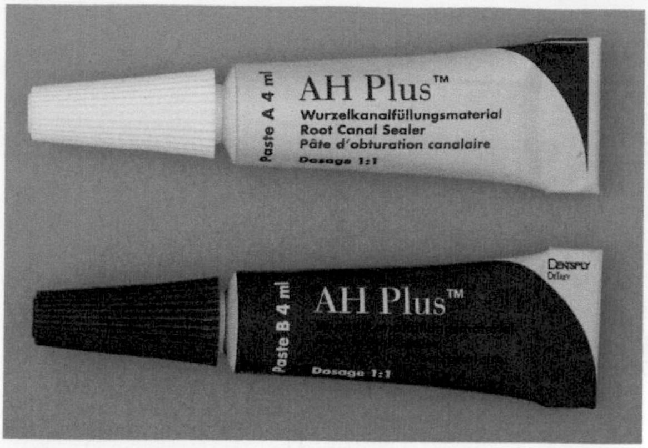

Figure 7.3 AH Plus root canal sealer.

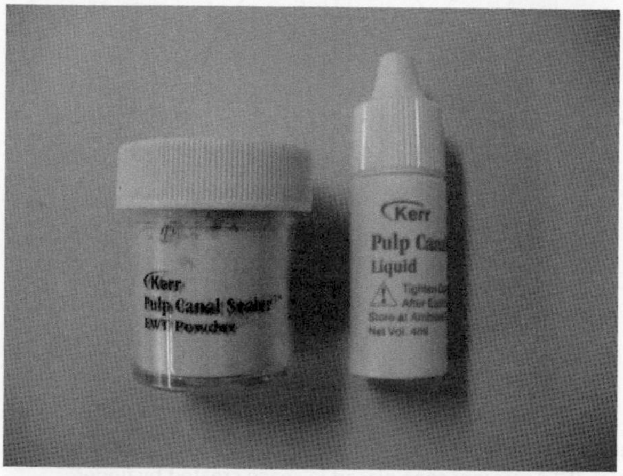

Figure 7.4 Pulp canal sealer.

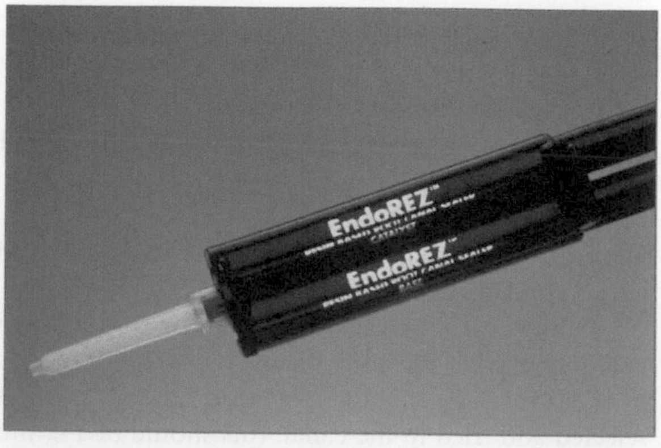

Figure 7.5 EndoREZ sealer.

which new techniques are compared. The objective is to fill the canal with gutta-percha points (cones) by condensing them laterally against the sides of the canal walls. The technique requires a tapered canal preparation, ending in an apical stop at the working length.

1. A spreader is selected that reaches to within 1 mm of the working length and the length marked with a rubber stopper. There are two main types of spreading instrument for condensing gutta-percha: long-handled spreaders and finger spreaders (Fig. 7.6A). The main advantage of a finger spreader is that it is not possible to exert the high lateral pressure that might occur with long-handled spreaders. The chance of a root fracture is reduced and it is therefore a suitable instrument for beginners.
2. A master point is selected that allows a friction fit in the apical portion of the root canal (Fig. 7.6B). When this is marked it is called 'tug back' (like pulling a dart out of a dart board). This may, however, be difficult to achieve with small size gutta-percha points, and therefore it is usual to accept a friction fit in narrow canals. A point, one size larger than the master apical file, is usually selected. If it is not possible to place the point to working length, select a point that passes to full length and trim 0.5 mm off the end using a scalpel (this has the effect of making the point slightly larger). Retry the point and adjust as necessary.
3. Mark the length of the point by nipping it with tweezers at the reference point and take a check radiograph with the cone in place.
4. Sealer placement: The sealer is mixed according to the manufacturer's instructions and introduced into the canal using a small sterile file rotated anticlockwise (omit this stage if there is a danger of sealer passing through the apical foramen, e.g. open apex). The master cone is then coated with sealer on the apical third and is introduced into the root canal slowly to aid coating of the canal walls and reduce the likelihood of sealer passing into the periapical tissues.
5. Once the master cone is seated, place a spreader between it and the canal wall, using firm pressure in an apical direction (Fig. 7.6C) (lateral pressure may bend or break the spreader or fracture the root). The spreader should pass to within 1 mm of

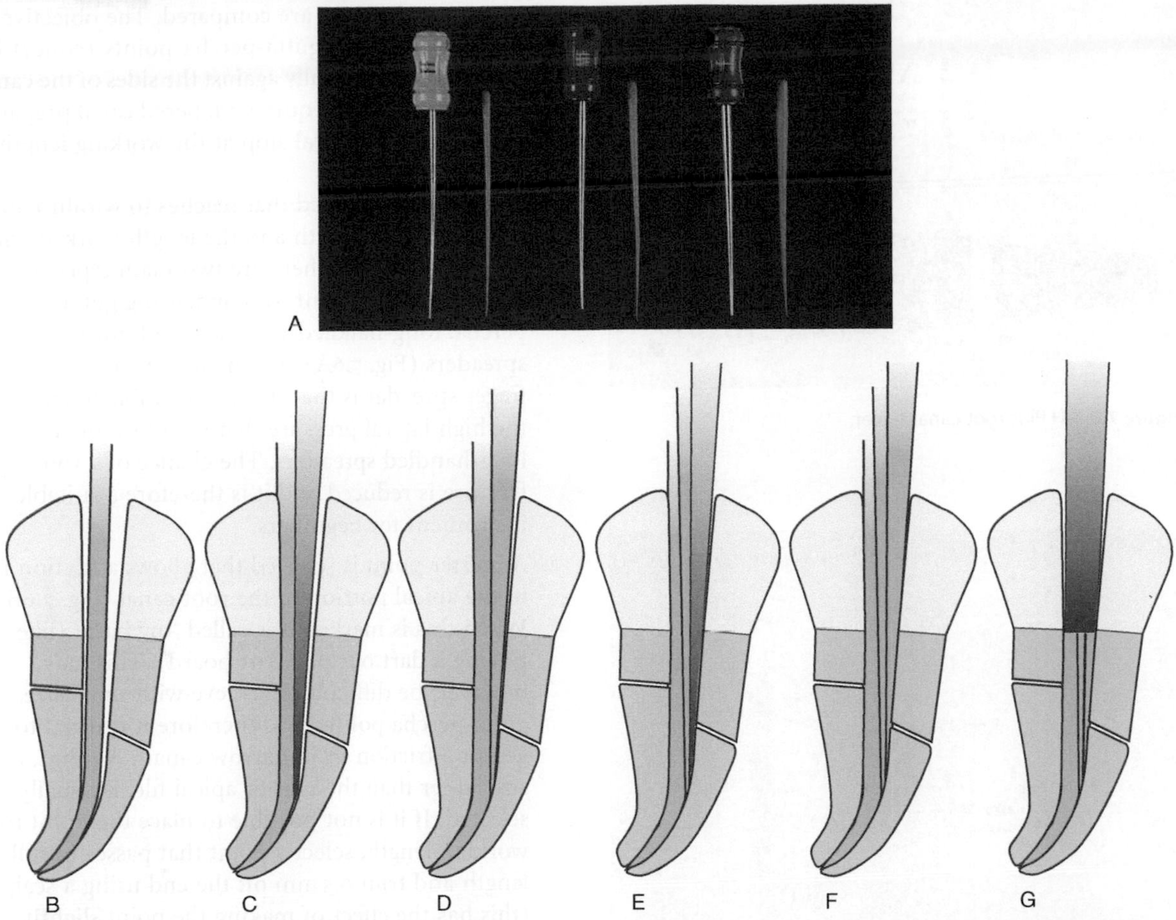

Figure 7.6 (A) Finger spreaders, size Fine Fine, Medium Fine and Fine with matching gutta-percha points. (B) Master gutta-percha point. (C) Finger spreader placed adjacent to master gutta-percha point. (D) Accessory cone placed in space created by finger spreader. (E–G) Spreaders and accessory cones placed to complete the obturation.

the working length.[5] This pressure, maintained for 20 seconds, will condense the gutta-percha apically and laterally, leaving a space into which an accessory point is placed.

6. An accessory cone the same size or one size smaller than the spreader is used. Rotate the spreader slightly, remove it, and immediately place the accessory cone (Fig. 7.6D). Repeat the procedure until the root canal is filled (Fig. 7.6E,F). The finger spreader condenses each cone into position; however, the final cone is not condensed as this would leave a spreader tract and contribute to leakage.
7. Cut off the gutta-percha 1 mm below the cement–enamel junction (CEJ) or gingival level, whichever is the more apical, using a hot instrument, and vertically condense the gutta-percha (Fig. 7.6G). This is important as remaining root filling material may stain the tooth.
8. If two or more canals are obturated with gutta-percha, undertake one at a time unless they meet in the apical third.
9. Seal the access cavity, remove the rubber dam and take a postoperative radiograph.

Figure 7.7 shows a clinical case of obturation with cold lateral condensation

In cases with apical resorption or complicated anatomy, the master cone may be adapted by the use of a solvent. A slightly oversized master cone is selected and tried in the canal; this should be 1–2 mm short of working length. The cone is removed and the

apical 2–3 mm briefly placed in a solvent (e.g. chloroform) for a maximum of 5 seconds (Fig. 7.8) and reintroduced into the canal; the procedure is repeated until the cone can be placed to working length. The cone is removed once the desired position is obtained, washed in alcohol to remove the solvent and placed in the canal with sealer. This is checked radiographically and, if satisfactory, the obturation is then completed with lateral or vertical condensation.

The cone may also be customized with a gauge (Fig. 7.9). This is particularly useful when a larger size cone is needed, and it may also be combined with a solvent to produce the desired size.

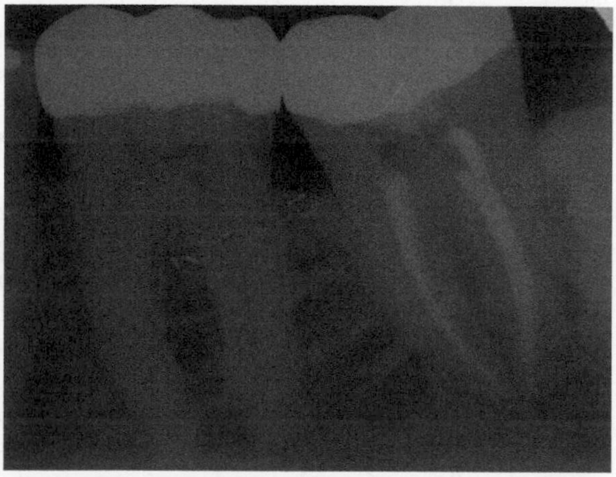

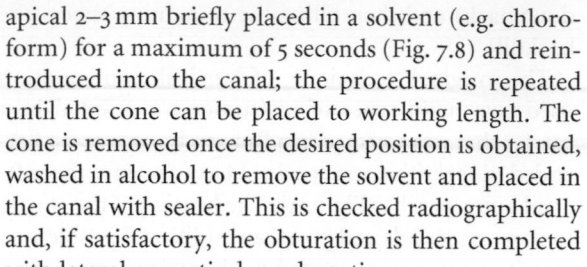

Figure 7.7 Obturation with lateral condensation.

Lateral condensation of warm gutta-percha

A modification to the cold lateral condensation technique is to perform it warm as this will soften the gutta-percha and make it easier to condense, possibly resulting in a denser root filling. The spreader may be heated by placing it in a hot bead sterilizer before insertion into the canal, although it should be emphasized that this is to provide heat for the spreader and

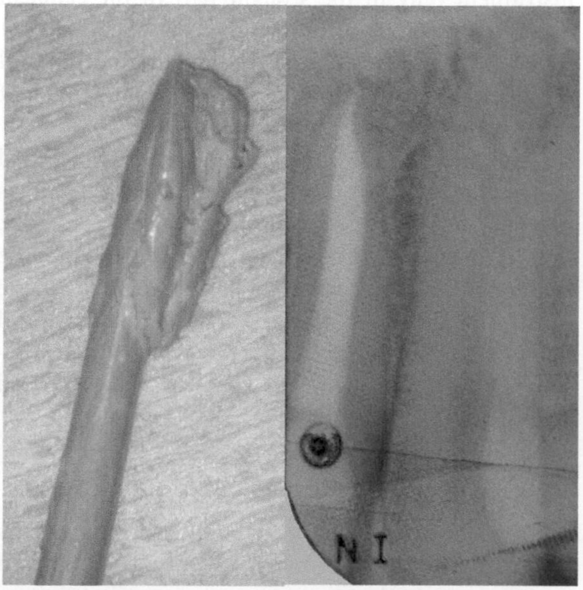

Figure 7.8 Gutta-percha point softened in chloroform and radiograph following vertical condensation.

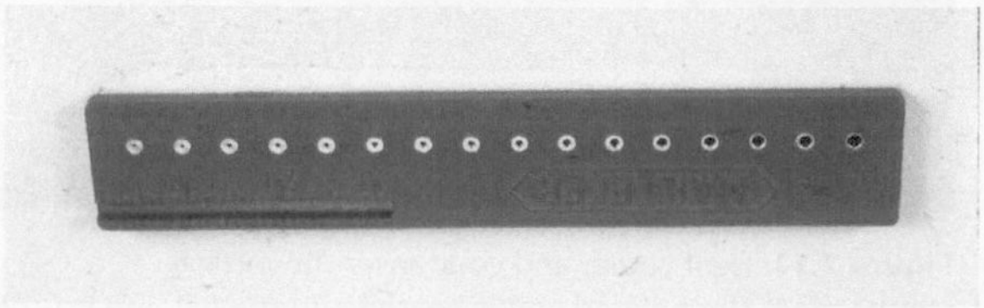

A

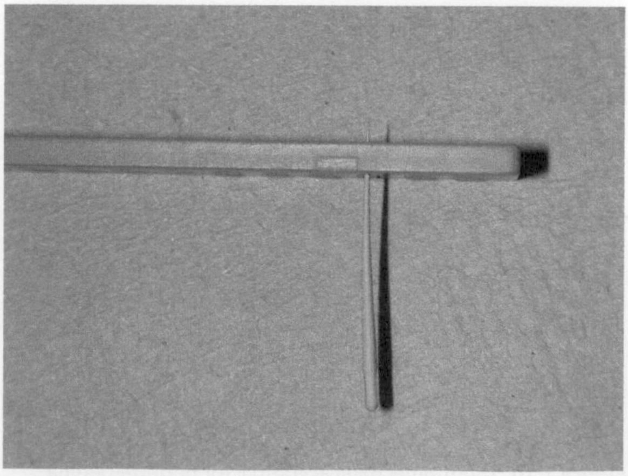

B

Figure 7.9 (A) Gauge for customizing a gutta-percha point. (B) Gutta-percha point being cut to the desired size.

is not an accepted method of sterilization. Alternatively, the friction of ultrasonic vibration may be used to introduce heat into the root filling.[3]

Lateral condensation and thermocompaction of gutta-percha

In this technique, a compactor which resembles an inverted file (Fig. 7.10) is placed in a slow-speed handpiece (8000 rpm) and used to help plasticize and condense the gutta-percha. Care must be taken to use this instrument only in the straight part of the canal in order to avoid gouging of the walls. The frictional heat from the compactor plasticizes the gutta-percha and the blades drive the softened material into the root canal under pressure.

A modification of the technique has been described as an adjunct to lateral condensation. Gutta-percha is first laterally condensed in the apical half of the canal, then a compactor is used to plasticize and condense the gutta-percha in the straight coronal half of the canal. The laterally condensed material in the apical half of the canal effectively prevents any apical extrusion and the softened gutta-percha is thus forced against the dentine walls.

Vertical condensation of gutta-percha

Thermal conductivity through gutta-percha occurs over a range of 2–3 mm and it only needs to be raised 3–8°C above body temperature (40–45°C) for it to become sufficiently mouldable. The requirements for vertical condensation of warm gutta-percha include a tapered preparation, accurate cone fit apically, suitable sealer, a heat source and a range of prefitted pluggers. Briefly, the technique of vertical condensation involves applying heat to the gutta-percha, condensing it down the root canal from coronal to apical (the downpack) and then filling the remaining space (the backfill).

The original technique of vertical condensation used two main types of instrument: a pointed heat carrier that was warmed in a Bunsen burner and a flat-ended plugger that was used cold to condense the softened gutta-percha (Fig. 7.11). The heating of the carrier took 5–10 seconds and posed an additional problem in that its temperature started to decrease as soon as it was removed from the flame, and consequently the carriers were heated until they were cherry-red hot; however, the recent introduction of electric heat carriers has enabled more control over the length of time the heat is applied.

Vertical condensation technique

The downpack is commenced by using the heat carrier to sear off the gutta-percha master cone at the canal orifice. Immediately following this, a cold plugger is introduced to condense around the periphery of the gutta-percha and seal the canal coronally. A sustained push is now applied to the centre of the gutta-percha, causing the sealer and warm gutta-percha to follow the path of least resistance down the main canal and along any lateral or accessory canals. This sustained push is termed a wave of condensation. The heat carrier is reapplied 3–4 mm into the gutta-percha and is removed with a small bite of gutta-percha attached. The filling is then condensed, as described above, to form a second wave of condensation. This cycle is repeated until 5 mm from the canal terminus, or to the end of the straight part of the canal, and a sustained

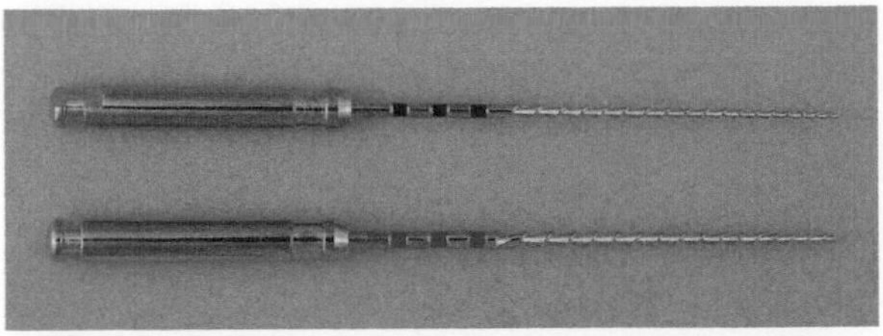

Figure 7.10 Thermomechanical compactor or gutta-percha condenser.

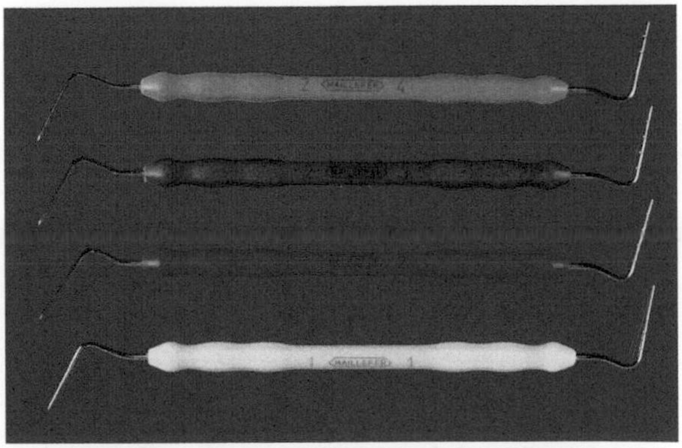

Figure 7.11 Heat carrier and condenser for vertical compaction. The pointed end is heated and the flat end is used cold for condensation.

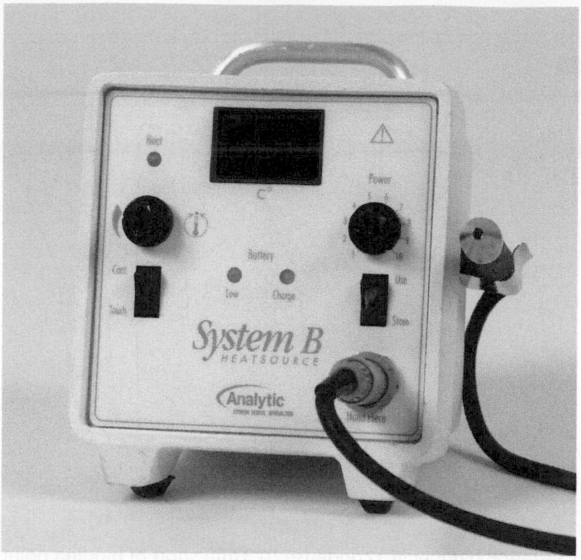

Figure 7.12 System B unit.

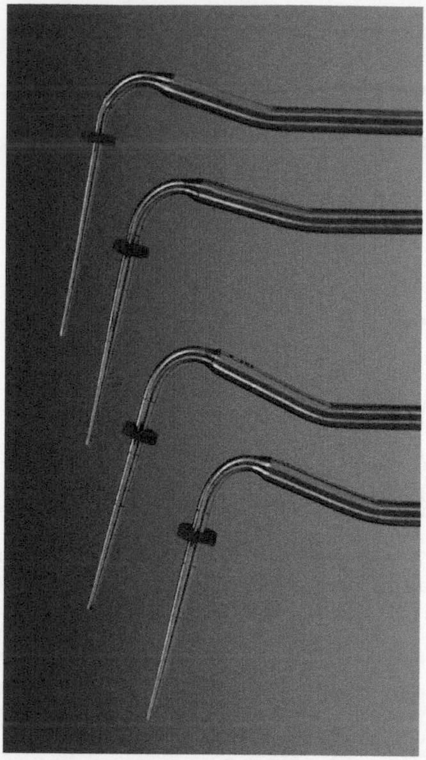

Figure 7.13 Buchanan pluggers for use with the System B unit.

application of apical pressure applied as the gutta-percha cools.

The downpack procedure results in apical corkage, filling of lateral and accessory canals and an empty canal space coronally. Backfilling of the canal is achieved by using thermomechanical condensation or thermoplasticized gutta-percha delivered in increments and condensed (see below). Vertical condensation produces excellent results in experienced hands, but has the problem of being time consuming.

Continuous wave of condensation

The 'continuous wave of condensation' has been introduced to further simplify and speed up vertical condensation. This technique uses a device, the System B (Fig. 7.12), which has four interchangeable soft steel pluggers: fine, fine medium, medium and medium large (Fig. 7.13). The pluggers are thermostatically controlled, can be heated to preset temperatures and maintain their temperature whilst condensing the gutta-percha within the root canal system. The appropriate plugger is selected to match the taper of the master cone, activated and used to condense the gutta-percha to just short of its binding point 5–7 mm from the terminus of the root canal, although it has been shown in vitro that the plugger must pass to within 3 mm of working length to heat the gutta-percha to the full length of the root canal.[6] The heat is then reactivated, the plugger drops to the binding point and is removed together with excess gutta-percha, providing an apical plug of gutta-percha.

In this technique the downpack consists of a continuous wave, rather than several interrupted waves of condensation. Backfilling can be achieved by using a series of gutta-percha points and thermomechanical compaction or ideally with the Obtura gun (see below). The continuous wave technique (Fig. 7.14) has been compared with a hybrid technique using multiple cones and was shown to be equally effective.[7]

The philosophy behind vertical condensation has not changed over three decades. The procedure aims to seal the terminus of the canal with an accurate cone fit and to pack the coronal end once the surplus gutta-percha has been removed. The downpack then forces sealer and gutta-percha along the lines of least resistance. Significant changes have been made in armamentarium, simplifying the technique and making it more operator friendly. Vertical condensation is, however, a taxing technique which, together with the expense of the initial purchase of the equipment,

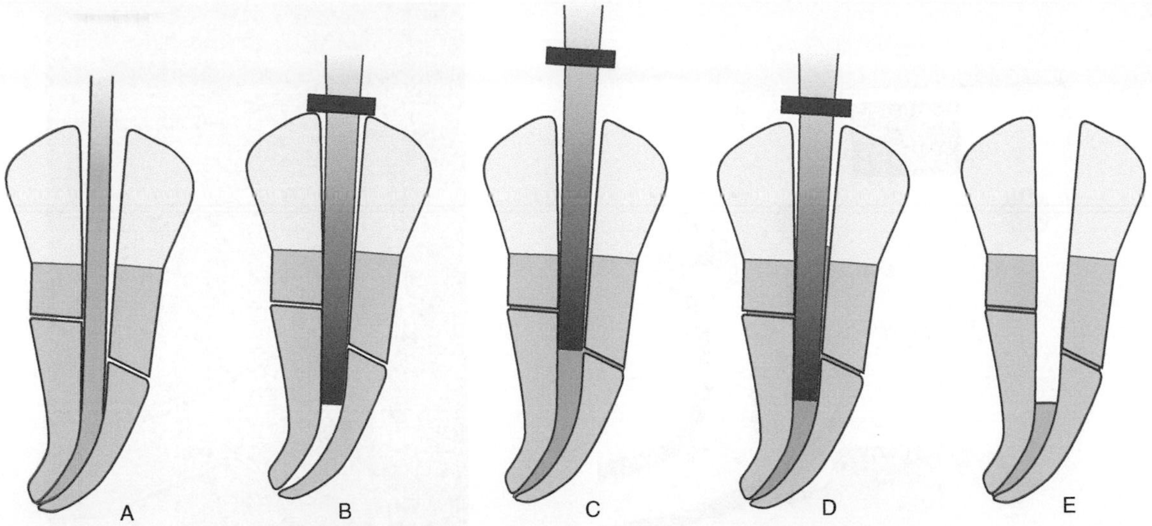

Figure 7.14 Continuous wave of condensation. (A) Cone fit; (B) try in System B plugger; (C) condense to 3 mm short of binding point; (D) separation burst after maintaining apical pressure for 10 seconds; (E) plugger removed and apical plug condensed by hand prior to back fill.

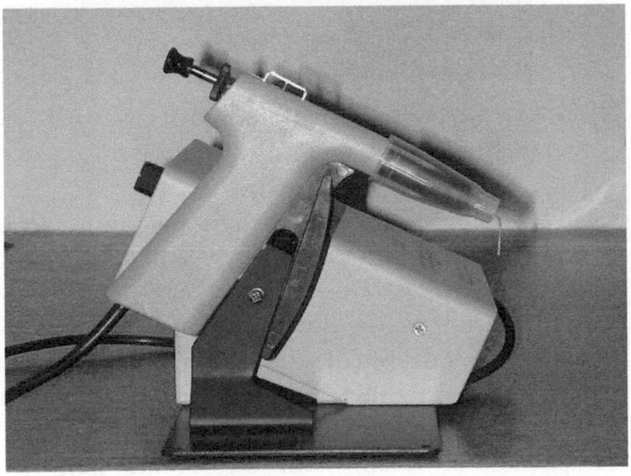

Figure 7.15 The Obtura unit.

probably explains the greater popularity of lateral condensation.

Thermoplasticized gutta-percha

The Obtura gun (Fig. 7.15), as used for the delivery of thermoplasticized gutta-percha, is particularly useful for backfilling during vertical condensation following creation of the apical plug. Small increments of gutta-percha are placed and condensed (Fig. 7.16) in order to keep shrinkage to a minimum. Examples of cases managed using the System B and Obtura are illustrated in Figure 7.17. The Obtura is also useful in cases of internal resorption, where the gutta-percha flows into canal irregularities as it is condensed (Fig. 7.18). Care must be taken to ensure that there is adequate

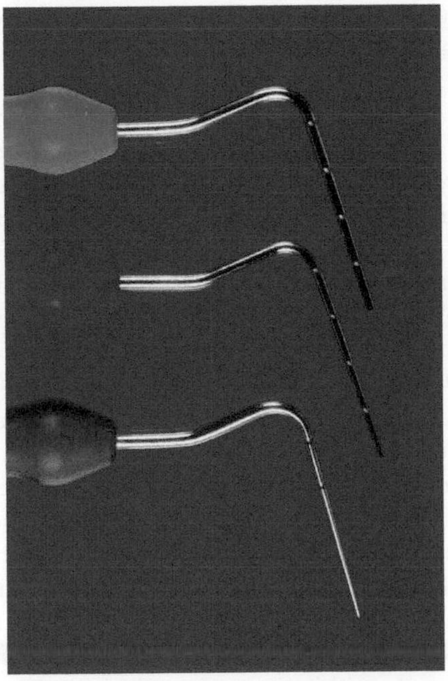

Figure 7.16 Vertical pluggers used in the backfill phase.

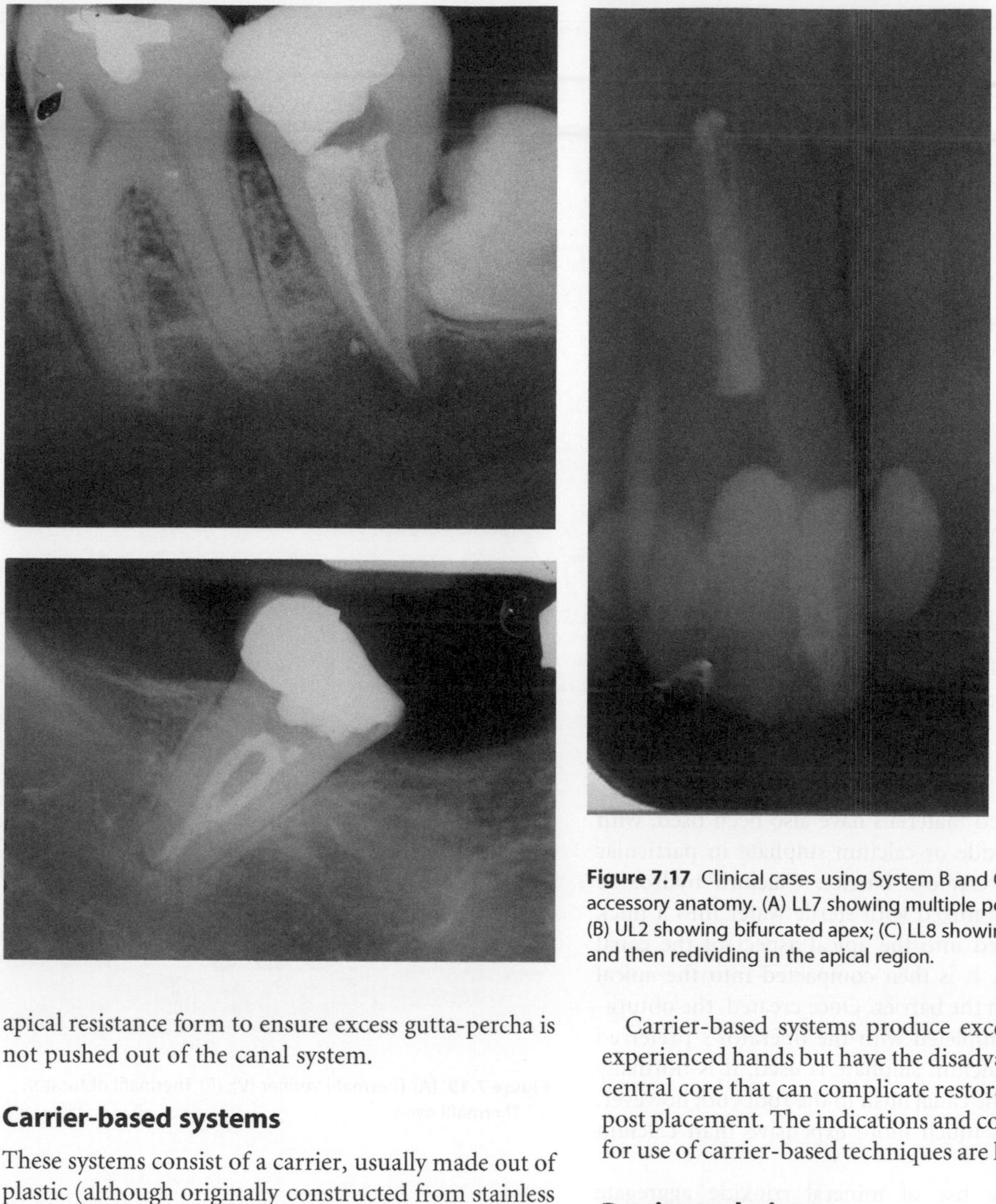

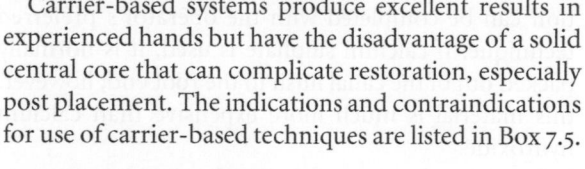

Figure 7.17 Clinical cases using System B and Obtura, noting accessory anatomy. (A) LL7 showing multiple portals of exit; (B) UL2 showing bifurcated apex; (C) LL8 showing canals fusing and then redividing in the apical region.

apical resistance form to ensure excess gutta-percha is not pushed out of the canal system.

Carrier-based systems

These systems consist of a carrier, usually made out of plastic (although originally constructed from stainless steel or titanium), which is supplied with a covering of gutta-percha. The size of the carrier required is checked using a size verification device (Fig. 7.19A). The appropriate carrier (Fig. 7.19B) is placed in the oven provided (Fig. 7.19C) and heated until the gutta-percha is soft. A small amount of sealer is placed in the canal and the carrier pushed home to the desired length. Additional condensation of the gutta-percha may be carried out adjacent to the carrier and the excess cut off in the pulp chamber at orifice level.

Carrier-based systems produce excellent results in experienced hands but have the disadvantage of a solid central core that can complicate restoration, especially post placement. The indications and contraindications for use of carrier-based techniques are listed in Box 7.5.

Barrier techniques

Certain situations may make the control of irrigating solutions and root filling materials difficult (e.g. a large apical foramen or open apex). In such situations, chlorhexidine may be used for apical irrigation and an apical barrier may be used to create a stop and control the obturation material. The use of dentine chips was reported many years ago although it does rely on the chips being uncontaminated by bacteria and their by-products.[8]

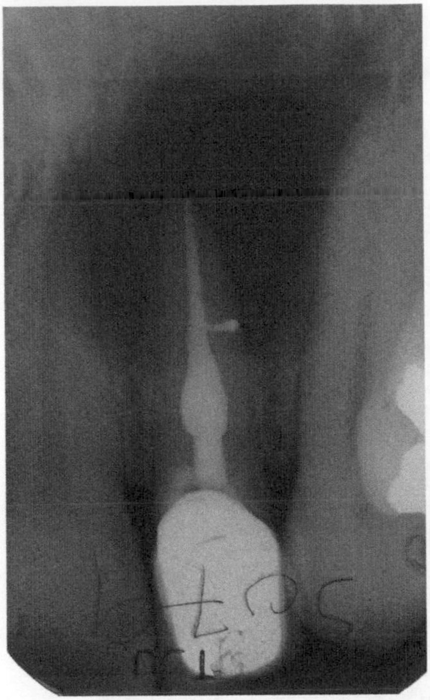

Figure 7.18 Use of Obtura in internal resorption.

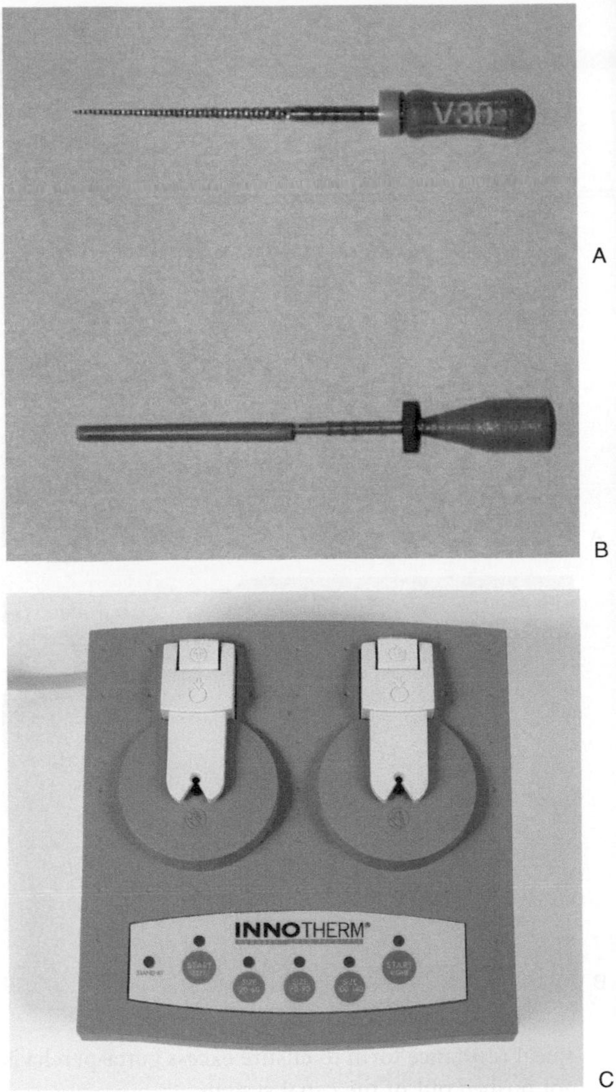

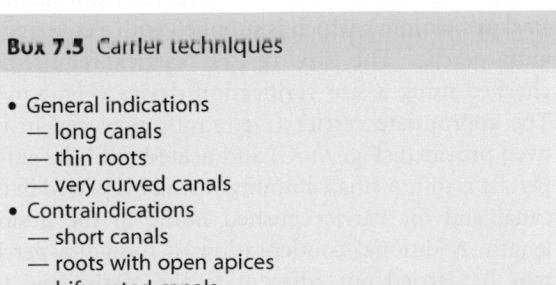

Figure 7.19 (A) Thermafil verifier (V); (B) Thermafil obturator; (C) Thermafil oven.

Calcium-based materials have also been used, with calcium hydroxide or calcium sulphate in particular being used to create a barrier. Calcium hydroxide powder may be mixed with sterile water into a thick paste and placed into the apical aspect of the canal using a carrier. It is then compacted into the apical 2–3 mm to form the barrier. Once created, the obturation can be completed with the operator's preferred technique. If calcium sulphate is used, it is normally packed out of the canal flush to the root end; however, this material is much more expensive than calcium hydroxide.

Recently, the use of mineral trioxide aggregate (MTA; Fig. 7.20) has been advocated for use in open apex cases with or without a barrier. It has the advantages of providing a good seal and being well tolerated by the apical tissues in that fibroblasts will attach to the material and the periodontal ligament fibres will regenerate. It requires a device for delivery into the canal (Fig. 7.21). A disadvantage, however, is that it has a long setting time, resulting in an additional appointment to confirm the material has set prior to the obturation being completed (Fig. 7.22).

Box 7.5 Carrier techniques

- General indications
  - — long canals
  - — thin roots
  - — very curved canals
- Contraindications
  - — short canals
  - — roots with open apices
  - — bifurcated canals

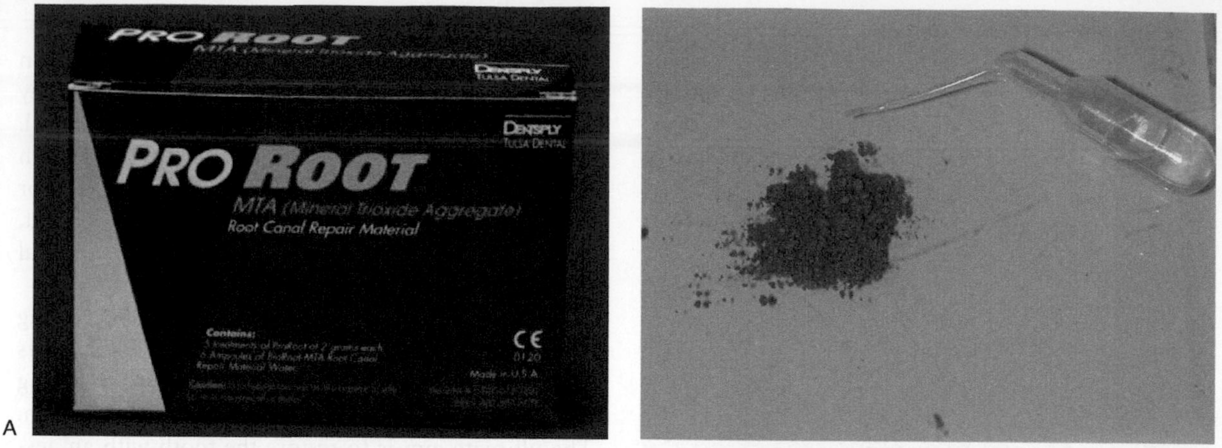

Figure 7.20 (A, B) Mineral trioxide aggregate.

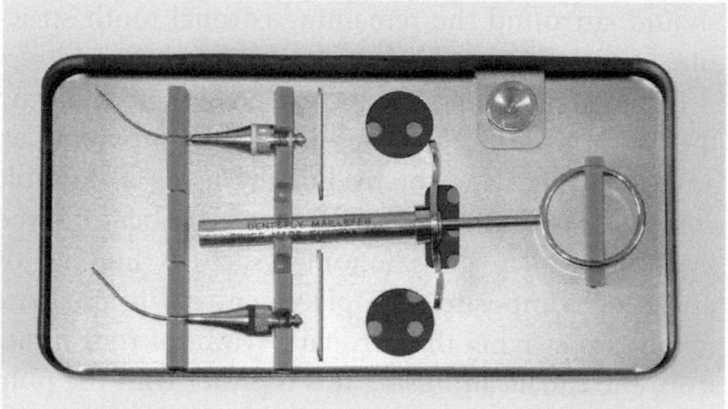

Figure 7.21 Carriers used for MTA placement.

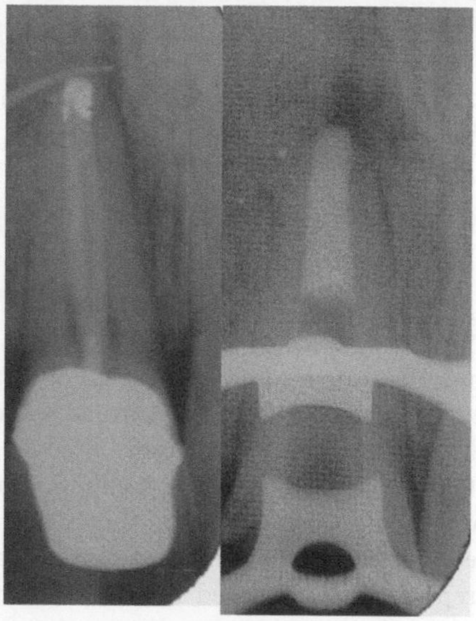

Figure 7.22 Retreatment case with MTA; the retrograde amalgam was delivered down the canal.

Overfills

Gutta-percha and root canal sealer may be extruded into the periradicular tissues during the obturation of the root canal system. Follow-up studies have shown that the success of treatment is lower when root canal materials are not confined to the root canal.[9] Where a solid piece of gutta-percha is extruded, a collagenous capsule is likely to form with minimal or no inflammation,[10] i.e. it is generally well tolerated by the tissues. However, small particles of gutta-percha can produce marked inflammation in the periradicular tissues.[11] A small amount of cement may be seen apically after obturation (Fig. 7.23), especially when using warm gutta-percha techniques. Large amounts of extruded root canal filling material may cause significant problems to the patient, especially if extruded into the inferior alveolar canal. Cement may also be seen opposite large accessory or lateral canals so it is important that a relatively inert sealer is used.

Proponents of vertical condensation argue the distinction between overfilling and vertical overextension of underfilled canal systems, i.e. filling materials may be overextended or extruded beyond a canal system that has not been sealed internally. Underfilling of a canal system could also indicate that it has not been debrided satisfactorily. In such situations necrotic pulp tissue, bacteria and their by-products would be expected to lead to failure. Overfilling infers that the whole canal system is obturated, but excess material

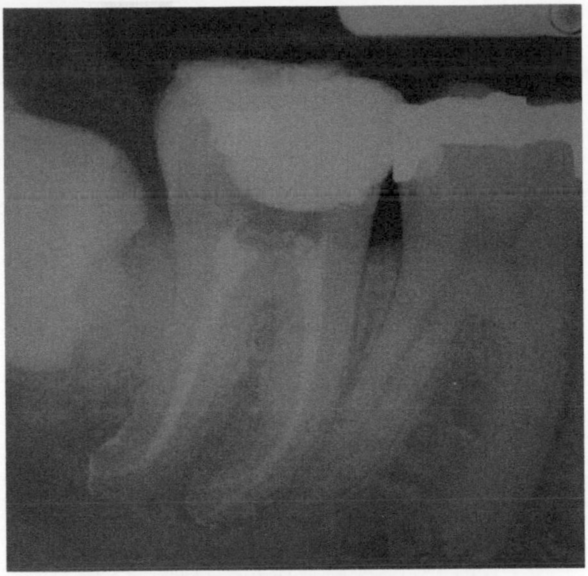

Figure 7.23 A small amount of sealer extruded through the apex seldom causes problems.

has been placed beyond the confines of the root canal and represents a quite different situation.

CORONAL SEAL

It is important after completing canal obturation to ensure that there is an adequate coronal seal over the root filling as coronal leakage has been shown to be an important cause of failure.[4] Clinically, findings have been ambivalent since one study shows that coronal leakage is perhaps not a significant cause of failure in well-prepared and obturated root canals,[12] but in a study where the majority of teeth were root filled and symptomatic with evidence of coronal leakage, a large number of bacteria have been isolated, the majority being Gram-positive facultative anaerobes.[13]

The coronal seal can be achieved by lining the floor of the pulp chamber with zinc oxide–eugenol cement or placing a layer of bonding resin or glass ionomer over the floor of the pulp chamber and canal orifices. In cases of post preparation, the apical gutta-percha can be sealed with zinc oxide–eugenol cement (Fig. 7.24); this is especially useful as temporary post crowns have a tendency to leak and may become decemented. It should be emphasized that an adequate seal is required in all aspects of the canal from the coronal to the apical; emphasis on one aspect of the canal should be avoided.

The rest of the seal

It is not the purpose of this text to discuss restoration of endodontically treated teeth; however, many aspects are critical to maintaining the coronal seal. Root canal treatment is performed on teeth with varying amounts of remaining tooth structure. If all or nearly all of the coronal tooth substance has been lost, then predictable long-term restoration and coronal seal may be problematic.

Successful restoration and seal rely on creating adequate resistance and retention form. This involves initial reinforcement and replacement of remaining tooth structure prior to an extracoronal restoration. The ultimate aim is to restore the tooth with an aesthetic restoration that is both biologically and mechanically sound. Ideally, this definitive restoration should surround the remaining coronal tooth structure, creating a reinforcing ferrule effect.

In molar teeth, it is frequently possible to build up the tooth, avoiding the use of posts, by providing an amalcore (Fig. 7.25) or by initially using a flowable composite over the floor of the pulp chamber followed by a resin-filled glass ionomer such as Fuji IX or posterior composite. The placement of an amalcore involves removing the coronal 2–3 mm of root filling from the canals and using this together with the pulp chamber to provide retention for the core build up. In anterior teeth, only the access cavity can be restored without resorting to posts, provided there is sufficient remaining tooth structure to support a veneer should aesthetics be a problem. The restoration of root-filled teeth, however, frequently involves the use of posts.

Post types

A vast array of different post types are available in different materials, together with a range of cements, both conventional (e.g. zinc phosphate) and, more recently, adhesive. It is essential to retain as much sound tooth structure as possible as this helps in reducing leverage forces in the root and potential fracture. Screw posts are not advocated as they create additional stresses in the root. Current opinion is that posts should fit passively in the canal and be used only if absolutely necessary. Although posts have traditionally been manufactured from metal, Composiposts used with adhesive cements are becoming increasingly popular with some operators.

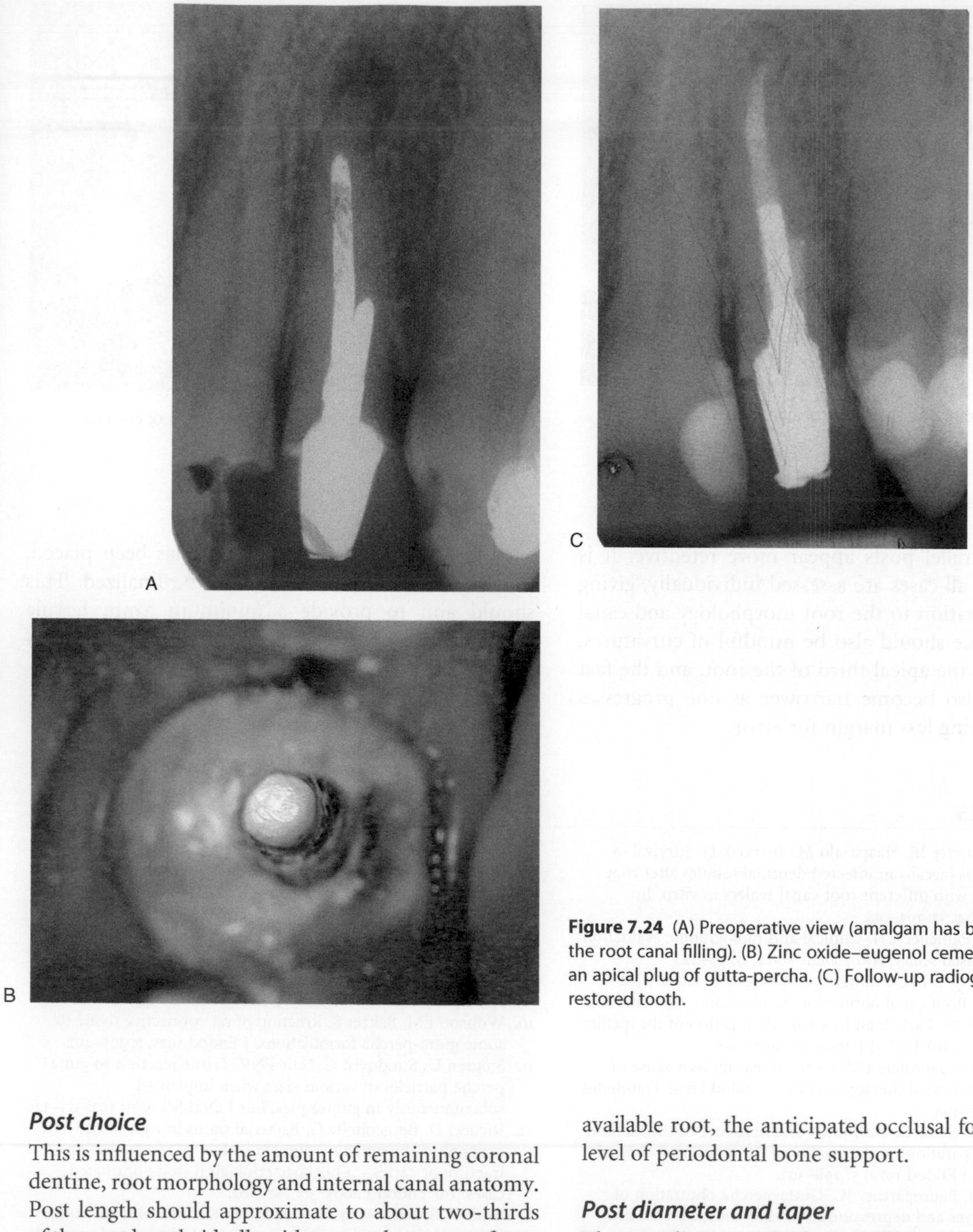

Figure 7.24 (A) Preoperative view (amalgam has been used as the root canal filling). (B) Zinc oxide–eugenol cement placed over an apical plug of gutta-percha. (C) Follow-up radiograph of restored tooth.

Post choice

This is influenced by the amount of remaining coronal dentine, root morphology and internal canal anatomy. Post length should approximate to about two-thirds of the root length, ideally with an equal amount of post below and above the alveolar crest. Care should be taken to leave an adequate amount of root canal filling material apically. Ideally this should be 5 mm; however, in short roots this may be reduced to 3.5 mm. Post length ultimately is affected by the length of the available root, the anticipated occlusal forces and the level of periodontal bone support.

Post diameter and taper

The post diameter ideally should not exceed the diameter of the optimally shaped and cleaned canal. A wider post does not mean more retention — post length is the more important factor.

Conflicting opinion exists as to post taper. Tapered posts are most compatible with root anatomy;

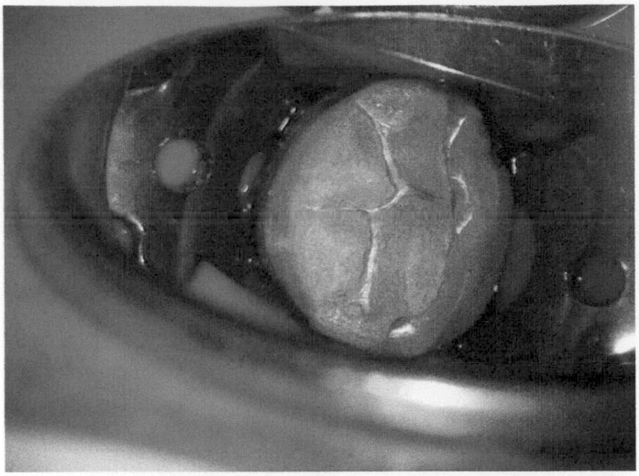

Figure 7.25 Example of an amalcore/amalgam onlay.

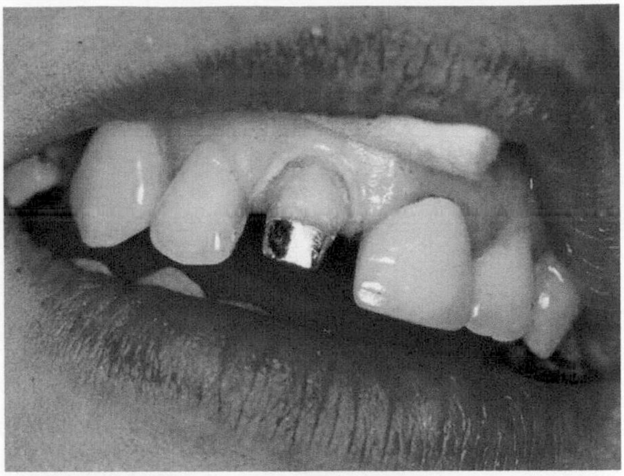

Figure 7.26 Anterior tooth showing retention of coronal dentine and a ferrule.

however, parallel posts appear more retentive. It is advised that all cases are assessed individually, giving due consideration to the root morphology and canal anatomy. One should also be mindful of curvatures, especially in the apical third of the root, and the fact that roots also become narrower as one progresses apically, leaving less margin for error.

Once an adequate core (± post) has been placed, then the coronal preparation can be finalized. This should aim to provide a minimum 2 mm ferrule around the coronal dentine to help prevent fracture of tooth structure (Fig. 7.26).

REFERENCES

1. Saleh IM, Ruyter IE, Haapasalo M, Ørstavik D. Survival of Enterococcus faecalis in infected dentinal tubules after root canal filling with different root canal sealers in vitro. Int Endod J 2004; 37: 193–198.
2. Zmener O, Pameijer CH. Clinical and radiographic evaluation of a resin based sealer. Am J Dent 2004; 17: 19–22.
3. Bailey GC, Ng Y-L, Cunnington SA, Barber P, Gulabivala K, Setchell DJ. Root canal obturation by ultrasonic condensation of gutta-percha. Part II: an in vitro investigation of the quality of obturation. Int Endod J 2004; 37: 694–698.
4. Saunders WP, Saunders EM. Coronal leakage as a cause of failure of root canal therapy: a review. Endod Dent Traumatol 1994; 10: 105–108
5. Allison D, Webber C, Walton R. The influence of the method of canal preparation on the quality of the apical and coronal obturation. J Endod 1979; 5: 298–302.
6. Bowman CJ, Baumgartner JC. Gutta-percha obturation of lateral grooves and depressions. J Endod 2002; 28: 220–223.
7. Guess GM, Edwards KR, Young ML, Iqbal MK, Kim S. Analysis of continuous wave obturation using single cone and hybrid techniques. J Endod 2003; 29: 509–512.
8. Holland R, De Souza V, Nery MJ, de Mello W, Bernabé CD, Otoboni Filho JA. Tissue reactions following apical plugging of the root canal with infected dentine chips. Oral Surg Oral Med Oral Path Oral Radiol Endod 1980; 49: 366–369.
9. Smith CS, Setchell DJ, Harty FJ. Factors influencing the success of conventional root canal therapy – a five year retrospective study. Int Endod J 1993; 26: 321–333.
10. Wolfson EM, Seltzer S. Reaction of rat connective tissue to some gutta-percha formulations. J Endod 1975; 1: 395–402.
11. Sjogren U, Sundqvist G, Nair PNR. Tissue reaction to gutta-percha particles of various sizes when implanted subcutaneously in guinea pigs. Eur J Oral Sci 1995; 103: 313–321.
12. Ricucci D, Bergenholtz G. Bacterial status in root filled teeth exposed to the oral environment by loss of restoration and fracture or caries – a histobacteriological study of treated cases. Int Endod J 2003; 36: 787–802.
13. Adib V, Spratt D, Ng YL, Gulabivala K. Cultivable microbial flora associated with persistent periapical disease and coronal leakage after root treatment: a preliminary study. Int Endod J 2004; 37: 542–551.

8 Root canal retreatment

Patients are becoming increasingly reluctant to loose teeth, which has led to the practitioner being faced with requests for retreatment of failing root canal treatment. Emphasis is frequently placed on mechanical problems that may have contributed to failure; however, the main aetiology is usually biological — the common factor being microorganisms — and thus it is important to understand their role in endodontic disease.

Causes of failure

A summary of reasons for failure of root canal therapy is outlined in Box 8.1. Frequent intraradicular causes include:

- necrotic material remaining in the root canal, either through failure to identify all canals or treating canals short
- contamination of an initially sterile root canal during treatment
- persistent infection of a root canal after treatment
- bacteria left in accessory or lateral canals
- loss of coronal seal and reinfection of a disinfected and sealed canal system.

Extraradicular causes of failure include persistent periradicular infection, radicular cysts and vertical root fractures.

Further causes of failure may be iatrogenic in nature, in particular when post space has been created without consideration being given to the internal and external root anatomy, with resultant perforation or root fracture.

Signs and symptoms of failure

These include a discharging sinus, pulpal pain or tenderness on biting. Frequently, however, symptoms may be absent with retreatment decisions being taken on incidental radiographic findings. For example, a periradicular radiolucency has appeared or increased in size following root canal therapy, or restorative treatment is proposed on a tooth without a lesion but with an apparently incompletely obturated root canal.

Treatment of failure

Failure, depending on its aetiology, is normally treated in one of three ways: root canal retreatment, periradicular surgery or extraction. Extraction is usually indicated for single rooted teeth with root fractures, unrestorable teeth and those with a hopeless periodontal prognosis. In multi-rooted teeth, it may be possible to resect a fractured or periodontally involved root, or to perform crown lengthening when gross caries is present, in order to make isolation and future restoration possible.

Recent developments in periradicular surgery are resulting in improved outcomes;[1] however, root canal retreatment is still normally considered preferable to surgical intervention, as the latter may seal over uncleaned canal space which could eventually leak. Further problems with a surgical approach include the effects of compromising root length and bone support on prosthetic or periodontal grounds. If, however, it is considered that access to the root canals cannot be gained without risk of compromising the tooth's prognosis or the financial implications of disassembly are prohibitive, then surgery is indicated.

ROOT CANAL RETREATMENT PROCEDURES

When infection is present the aim of root canal retreatment is to eliminate microorganisms that have either survived previous treatment or have re-entered the root canal system. The feasibility of retreatment depends on the operator's ability to gain access to the root canal system, in particular the apical third. Careful assessment of the preoperative radiograph should be made with regard to whether or not a post

Box 8.1 Reasons for failure of root canal treatment

Intraradicular

- Bacteria and necrotic material remaining in the root canal following initial treatment
- Untreated or undertreated canals
- Contamination of an initial sterile root canal during treatment through poor asepsis
- Bacteria remaining after treatment
- Loss of coronal seal and reinfection

Extraradicular

- Persistent periradicular infection
- Radicular cysts
- Root fracture

Iatrogenic

- Post perforation

Box 8.2 Stages of root canal retreatment

- Coronal access
- Radicular access
- Removal of root filling materials
- Negotiation of blocked or ledged canals, regaining canal patency
- Preparation of the canal
- Antimicrobial management
- Obturation and restoration

has been used, what type it is, the type of root filling material (paste, gutta-percha, silver point) and potential problems such as curves, perforations or ledges. The stages of root canal retreatment are outlined in Box 8.2.

Access to the pulp chamber and root canal system is usually complicated by the presence of coronal restorations, retentive devices and obturation materials. The use of additional magnification and lighting is especially useful in root retreatment procedures. Loupes and a headlamp will provide good visibility of the pulp chamber floor and canal orifices. Working in the middle and apical thirds of the root canal, however, requires the use of the operating microscope[2] to see clearly.

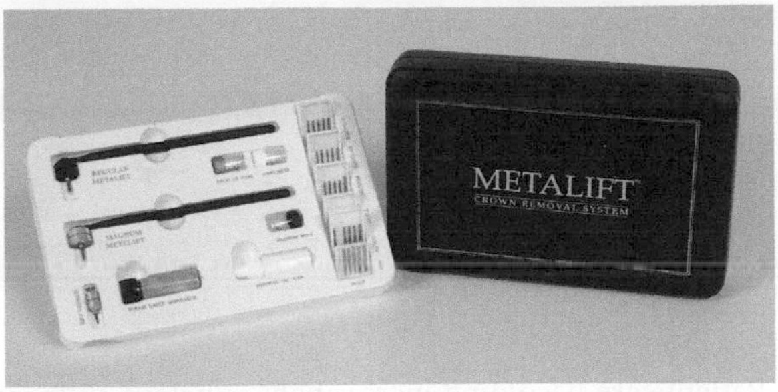

Figure 8.1 Metalift system. A small hole is drilled in the occlusal surface of the restoration prior to the introduction of a self-threading screw which pushes against the dentine/core and elevates the crown, thus breaking the cement seal.

Coronal access

Careful consideration should be given to the quality of the coronal restoration prior to access. Where the coronal restoration is satisfactory, it should be retained and access made through it, with due care and attention given to bur angulation as the original coronal landmarks of the tooth may have been lost. The presence of an integral post and core or evidence of leakage around the restoration margins usually indicates that it should be removed prior to performing root canal retreatment.

Sectioning and removal of crowns or bridges, with careful consideration being given to the method of temporization, is to be preferred to tapping them off with a crown remover. The latter method is uncontrolled and may result in unnecessary fracture of tooth tissue, with subsequent restorative complications. It is advisable to initiate sectioning with a diamond bur if porcelain is involved, otherwise the transmetal bur provides an excellent means of cutting through metal crowns. A recent device, the Metalift (Fig. 8.1), has been introduced, which allows crowns to be removed intact. The procedure involves drilling a small hole in the occlusal surface of the restoration prior to the introduction of a self-threading screw which pushes against the dentine/core and elevates the crown, thus breaking the cement seal.

On occasion, it may be possible to seal leaking restorations internally as a temporary measure to exclude bacteria and prevent leakage of irrigation solutions. Removal of the restoration, however, has the advantages of ensuring removal of all caries, allows a thorough check to be made for cracks and provides

excellent access for identifying previously untreated canals. In cases of extensive breakdown, it may be necessary to place a copper ring (Fig. 8.2) or orthodontic band and build a restoration, prior to embarking on treatment in order to ensure a seal around the margins of the rubber dam, avoid compromising asepsis and provide a four-walled access cavity for containing irrigant solutions.

Radicular access, removal of restorative materials

Once coronal access has been gained then attention is addressed towards radicular access. Core materials will either be tooth or non-tooth coloured materials or cast metal. The most common non-tooth coloured material is amalgam which can be removed superficially using surgical length round tungsten carbide burs in the high-speed handpiece, followed by long neck burs used at slow speed deeper in the access cavity. When the floor of the pulp chamber is approached, ultrasonic tips (Fig. 8.3) offer a safer alternative, compared to burs, for dispersing any material remaining over furcal areas and in the orifices of root canals. Tooth coloured cores may be more difficult to distinguish from dentine and careful observation of the dried access cavity floor, to differentiate between dentine and restorative material, is important, as is tactile exploration with an endodontic explorer. The access cavity should be re-evaluated at this stage, in regard to its extent, to look for previously untreated canals and ensure files are able to pass into the canal without touching the walls. Such interferences may result in small amalgam filings being created which can pass apically and block the canal.

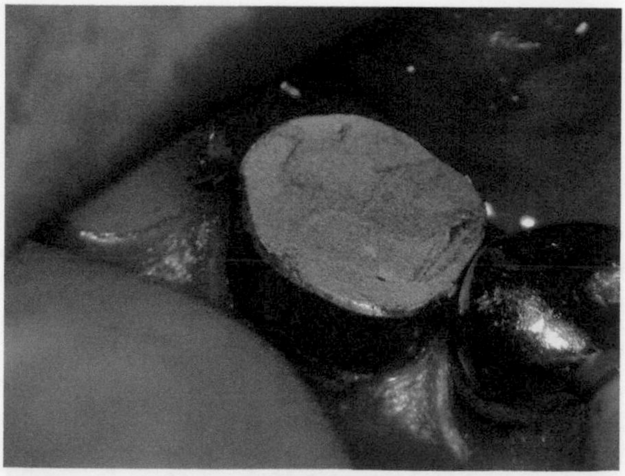

Figure 8.2 Tooth restored with copper ring and amalgam prior to root retreatment. Composite or resin reinforced glass ionomer or orthodontic bands may also be used.

Radicular access, removal of post and cores

Post and core build ups may be all-in-one castings or a combination of preformed posts and plastic core materials. In the latter cases the core should be dissected away in order to expose the individual posts.

The removal of a post should not be attempted if the force to remove it could result in root fracture. Ultrasonic vibration may be used initially to try to break the cement seal. The vibrations should be directed in a coronal direction, which necessitates the cutting of a notch on the side of the core. If a specialized tip is not available then a standard ultrasonic scaler may be used. Care must be taken with ultrasonic vibration, as heat is produced which can cause local bone necrosis. It is therefore important to use coolant water spray, intermittent application and moderate power, as high settings may initiate microcracks in the root. In some situations, ultrasonic vibrations may result in the post becoming free within the canal; however, if it does not, then it is necessary to use a device to extract the post and core. This can usually be accomplished in anterior teeth using the Ruddle post removal system (Fig. 8.4) which consists of a series of trepans to mill the post, tubular taps to engage the post and extraction pliers to provide the elevation force.

Recent developments have seen changes in post technology, in particular the use of cements to bond posts into place and those fabricated out of alternative materials, such as composite or fibre posts whose radiopacity may resemble gutta-percha. Metal posts cemented with composite cements can be extremely difficult to remove, especially if they are of sound design. Such difficulties are likely to increase in the future and may see an increase in periradicular surgery. Composite or fibre posts normally pose less of a challenge and frequently can be removed using ultrasonic vibration or drilling. It is important to make a note of the type of post and cement used in the patient record, as such information is then available to inform decision making in the future.

The fracture of a post within a root canal can pose a major problem and care should be taken to try not

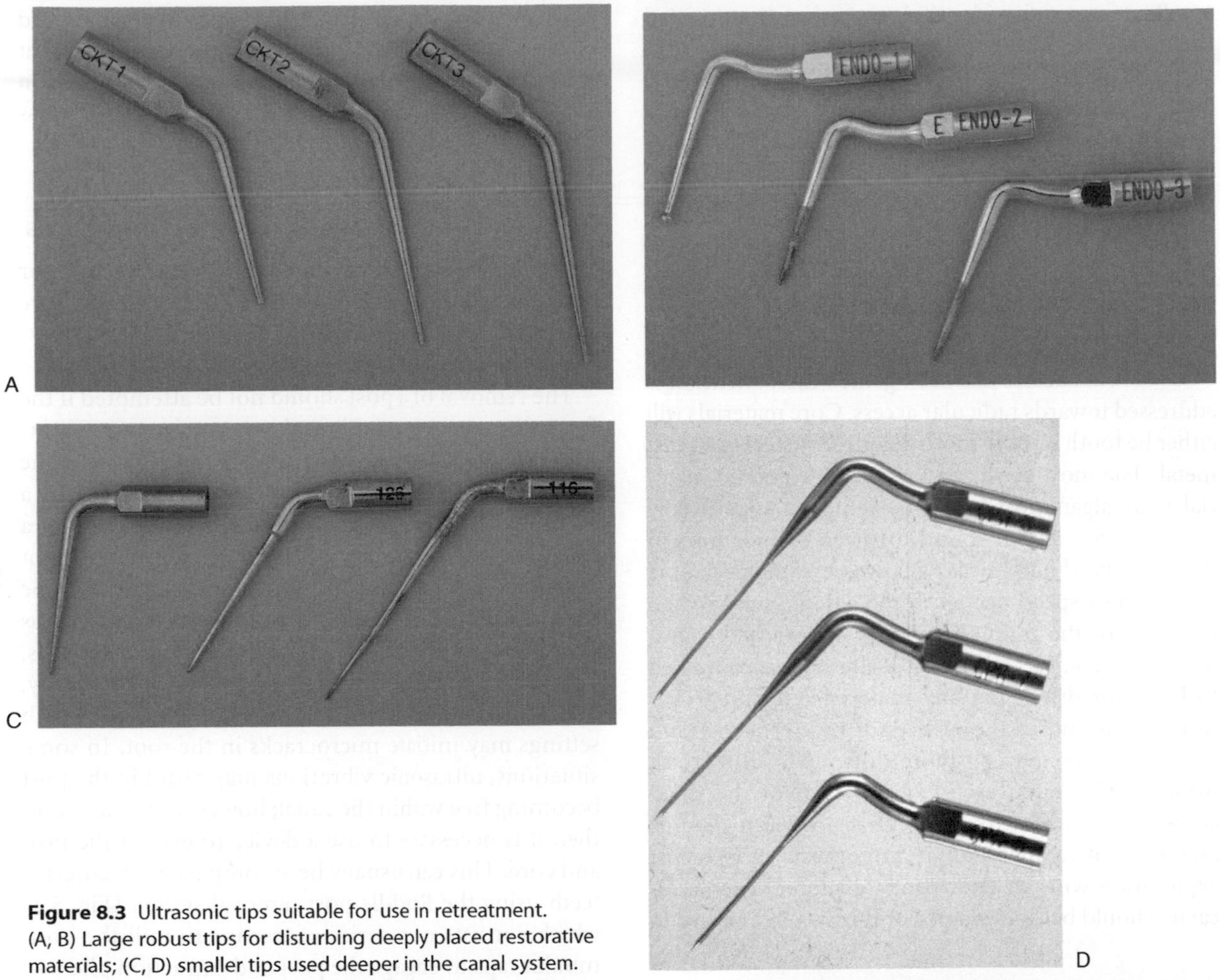

Figure 8.3 Ultrasonic tips suitable for use in retreatment. (A, B) Large robust tips for disturbing deeply placed restorative materials; (C, D) smaller tips used deeper in the canal system.

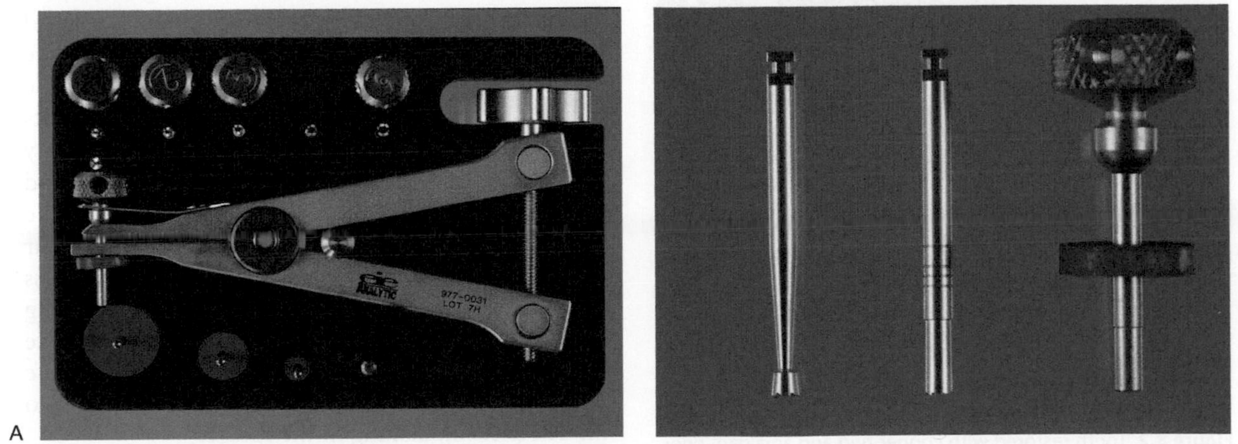

Figure 8.4 (A) The Ruddle post removal system including the extractor. (B) A domer bur, trepan and tap used to modify and engage the post.

to further weaken, fracture or perforate the root. Such situations should first be tackled by troughing around the post to remove the luting cement, using a small long neck bur or thin ultrasonic tip (Fig. 8.5).

Use of ultrasonic tips will remove many fractured posts without having to resort to additional means, such as the Masserann kit (Fig. 8.6). The Masserann system is preferred to the Ruddle for removal of fractured posts, as the metal trepans are thinner and therefore more conservative of tooth tissue. A suitably sized trepan is directed along the side of the post in the space

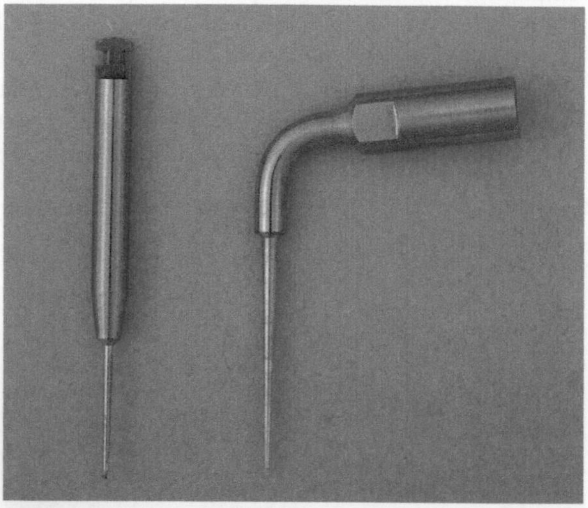

Figure 8.5 An LN bur and small ultrasonic tip showing comparison in size.

created by the ultrasonic tips. A smaller trepan may then be used to grip and remove the fractured portion (additional ultrasonic vibration applied to the trepan may be useful at this point). If the post is of the screw-in type, then it may be unscrewed after the use of ultrasound to weaken the cement seal, either by placing a groove in its end or grasping it with a tight-fitting trepan. If this is unsuccessful, then a trepan should be selected which will cut along the threads of the post, as this will minimize the amount of dentine removed while easing the cutting of the metal. In exceptional cases, fractured posts may be drilled out using an end-cutting bur. This procedure, however, is rarely necessary in view of the recent developments in ultrasonic tip design and improved magnification and lighting.

Access to the apical third

Access to the apical third of the root is usually restricted by the presence of materials used to obturate the canal (Box 8.3). Those most frequently used include pastes, gutta-percha and silver points. A thorough evaluation of the access cavity should be performed, modifying it as necessary to give straight line access to the root canals prior to attempting removal of the obturation materials.

Removal of pastes

Soft pastes can usually be easily penetrated using short sharp hand files and copious irrigation. The use of an

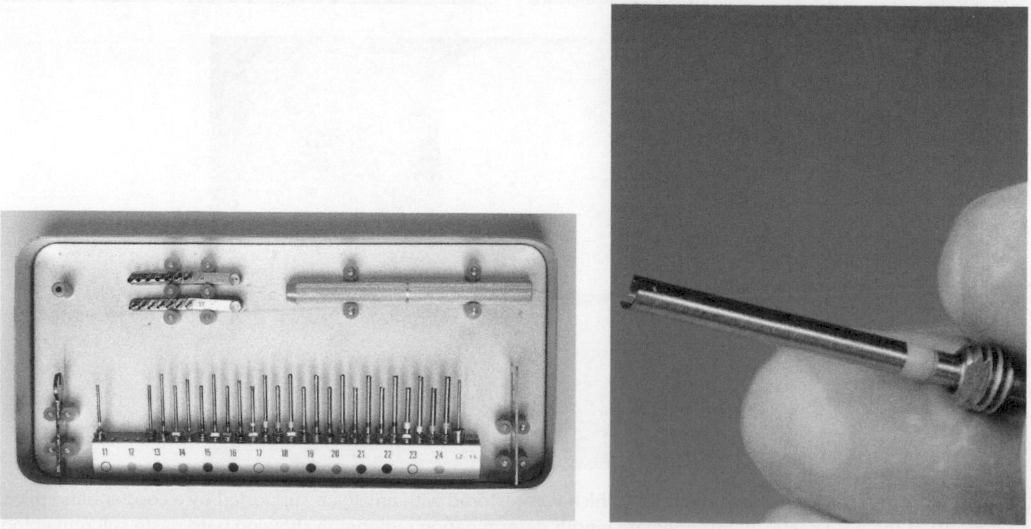

A

B

Figure 8.6 (A) Masserann kit. (B) Close-up of a Masserann trepan.

ultrasonically powered file, with accompanying irrigation, can be helpful in these situations, especially for removing remnants of paste from root canal walls, which may remain despite careful hand instrumentation. It is important to remove such remnants, as they block tubules, fins, etc., preventing the dentine surface from being exposed to irrigating solutions. Rotary nickel titanium (NiTi) instruments may also be used to help in removal, but only after a smooth glide path has been established with hand files.

Hard pastes can be particularly difficult to remove and usually need to be drilled out with a small long neck bur or chipped out using an ultrasonic insert, as described previously. These procedures can only be used in the straight part of the canal and it is important to use magnification and lighting, as they are high risk and can lead to going off line and perforation. Irrigation with ethylenediaminetetraacetic acid (EDTA) and sodium hypochlorite (NaOCl) should be employed, together with frequent drying, to ensure good visibility, especially deep within the canal. Small files may also be used and penetration can sometimes be achieved, as paste root fillings tend to be denser coronally and do not always set fully in the apical part of the root canal (Fig. 8.7). Mixed results may be

Box 8.3 Common types of obturating material

- Pastes, soft or hard
- Gutta-percha
- Silver points, full length or sectional
- Carrier-based materials

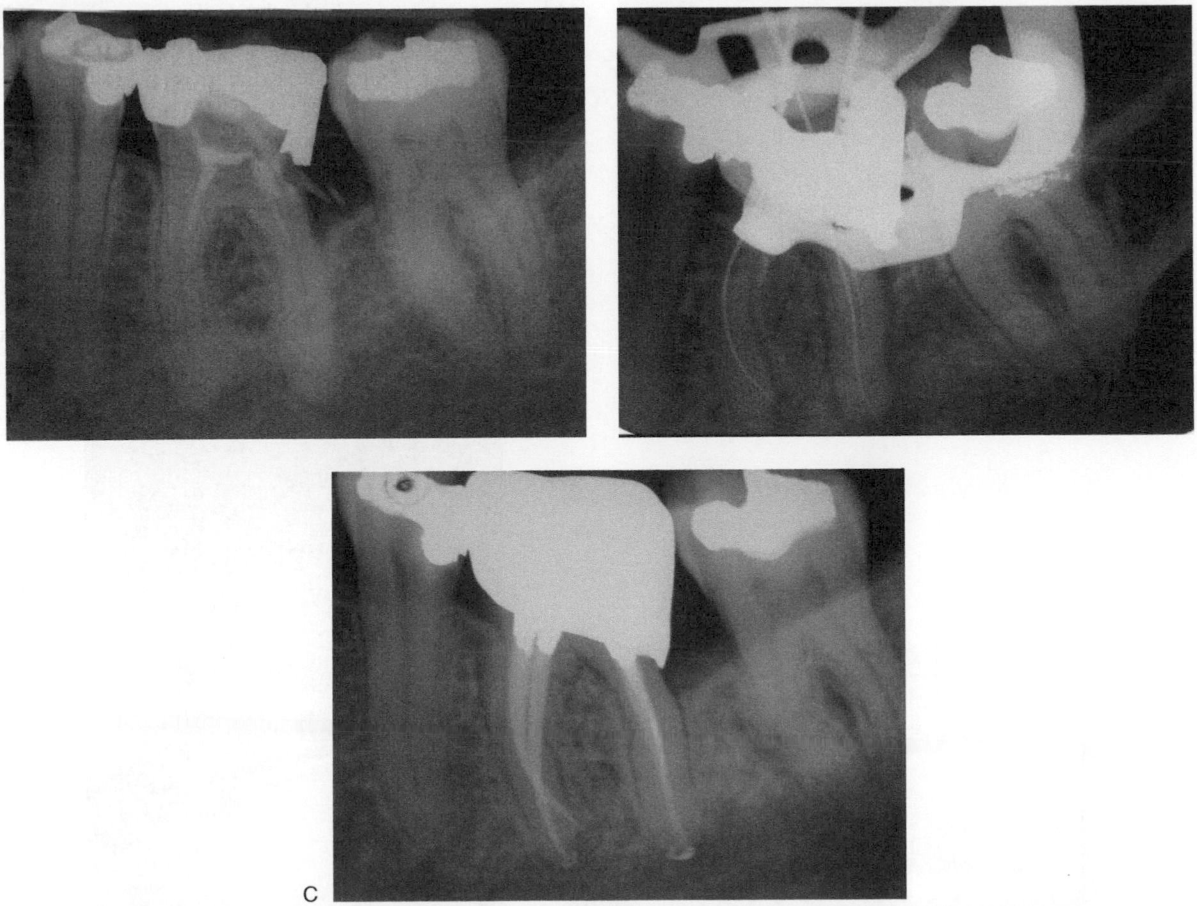

A B C

Figure 8.7 (A) A badly broken down lower first molar which was restored with amalgam supported by a copper band prior to attempting removal of the hard paste. (B) Intermediate length determination radiograph showing hard paste still remaining deep within two of the canals. This was removed using an LN bur and ultrasonics. (C) Amalgam core and coronal restoration in place.

obtained with solvents such as chloroform, Endosolv-E or Endosolv-R.

Removal of gutta-percha

Gutta-percha root fillings, which have been inadequately laterally condensed, may be removed by rotating one or two small Hedstrom files around or between the root canal filling points, pulling and elevating the points intact. An attempt should always be made to remove overextended points intact, as once solvents are used it becomes more difficult to grasp the point and remove overextended material. If this is unsuccessful, then removal of the root canal filling should be considered in stages, removing first the coronal, followed by the middle and apical thirds.

Gates-Glidden burs may be used coronally in the straight part of appropriately sized canals. These are available in a range of sizes and have a safe cutting tip that reduces the risk of perforation, providing too large a size is not used. Care should be taken during their use, as if too fast a speed is used then they may inadvertently screw into the canal and cause considerable damage; a suitable speed is 1000–1500 rpm. Other rotary instruments that may be used for the removal of gutta-percha include those made from nickel titanium (e.g. ProFiles or Orifice Shapers). These instruments are useful for removing coronal gutta-percha from large canals and around curves, provided a glide path has been confirmed. They are used at a higher speed (up to 500 rpm, in the straight part of the canal, to soften and elevate gutta-percha) than that used for canal preparation. Care is needed, however, when advancing around curves or into the apical region, when the speed should be reduced to 300 rpm.

Heat may be used to soften and remove gutta-percha in narrow canals, followed by files and solvent. Once a curvature is approached then it is important to use a solvent such as chloroform, oil of cajeput or oil of turpentine to soften the gutta-percha, aid mechanical removal and reduce the chance of transporting the main axis of the canal. Chloroform is the most effective solvent for dissolving gutta-percha.[3,4] A small drop placed in the canal is all that is required, as it softens only the coronal end of the gutta-percha, which is then removed with hand files. The chloroform is replaced frequently as softened gutta-percha is removed and progress made to the terminus of the canal. Gutta-percha, softened with chloroform, tends to smear the canal walls; this can be removed by paper point wicking. However, since chloroform itself — like all solvents — has a potentially toxic effect, it is important to use it sparingly.

Removal of silver points

Silver points are round in cross-section and therefore rarely seal canals adequately. Leakage occurs when sealer washes out, with subsequent corrosion leading to failure of the root canal filling. The approach to removal depends on whether the point extends and can be seen to extrude within the pulp chamber. In such situations silver point snugness should be assessed by grasping with Steiglitz forceps (Fig. 8.8)

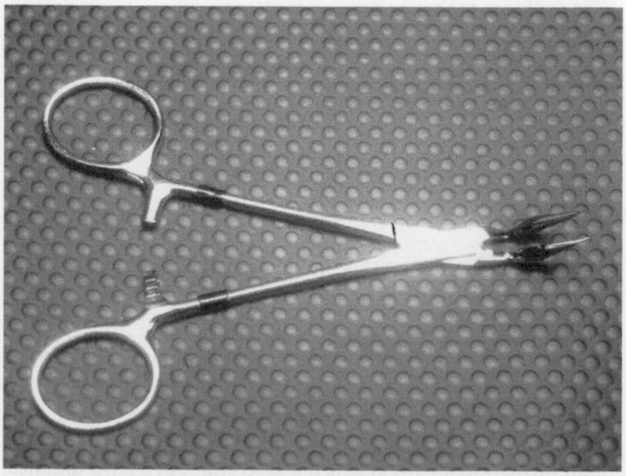
A

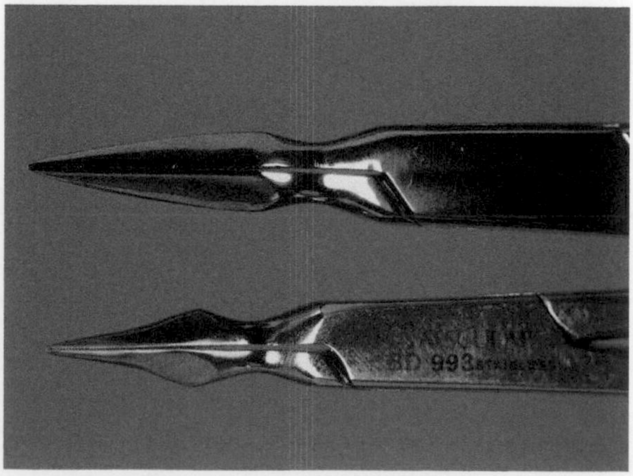
B

Figure 8.8 Steiglitz forceps (A) before and (B) after modification on a prosthetics lathe.

and levering gently, using the coronal aspect of the tooth as a fulcrum. Loose points will be easily removed in this manner and gentle manipulation is unlikely to remove valuable coronal silver points, which may be required for future grasping and extraction attempts. If the points cannot be removed easily, then ultrasonic vibration can be applied to the forceps holding the point.

If the silver point has been cut off at the canal orifice, then it is usually not possible to grip it. In such situations an ultrasonic tip may be used to cut a trough around the point. Care needs to be taken not to touch the point, as the silver is much softer than the steel used for manufacture of the ultrasonic tip, and preferential removal of the point will occur. A variety of removal techniques may be employed to grip the point and remove it once a trough approximately 2 mm deep has been prepared, such as a Masserann extractor (Fig. 8.9A), Ruddle IRS (Fig. 8.9B) or tube and glue/composite (see 'Management of fractured instruments',

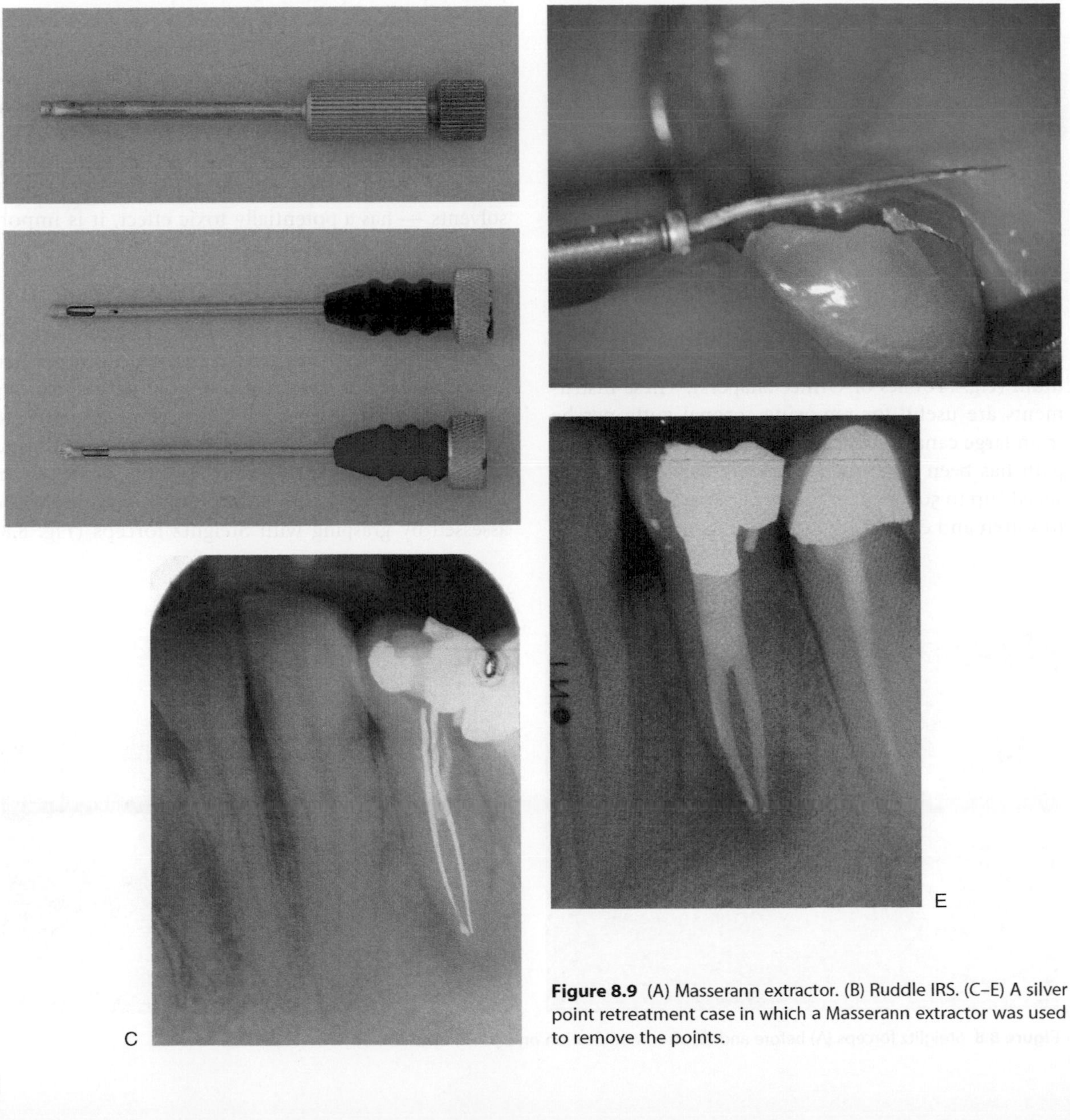

A B C D E

Figure 8.9 (A) Masserann extractor. (B) Ruddle IRS. (C–E) A silver point retreatment case in which a Masserann extractor was used to remove the points.

below). A silver point retreatment case is illustrated in Figure 8.9(C–E).

On occasion it may be necessary to work a size 15 ultrasonic file down the side of a point placed deep in a root canal. Removal in these situations may be facilitated by placing a Hedstrom file alongside the point to aid elevation, with or without ultrasonic vibration.

Removal of carriers

Carrier obturation techniques consist of a core surrounded by gutta-percha, and a combination of techniques used for the removal of gutta-percha and silver points is frequently indicated. Initial exploration along the side of the carrier with a solvent will remove gutta-percha, create space in larger canals and may locate a groove on the side of the carrier to pass a rotary NiTi file alongside and frequently elevate the point. If this is not successful, then grasping or elevation techniques (as described in 'Removal of silver points', above) may be employed (Fig. 8.10).

MANAGEMENT OF FRACTURED INSTRUMENTS

Instrument fracture can occur during root canal preparation but is not a negligent act; however, not informing the patient of such an event would constitute negligence. Key factors in minimizing instrument fracture are outlined in Box 8.4.

Stop and evaluate

The first thing to do in the event of a fractured instrument is to stop and evaluate the situation, as fractured instruments themselves are not a direct cause of failure, rather it is the indirect effects they may have,

Box 8.4 Key considerations in minimizing instrument fracture

1. Considering files as disposable items, discarding damaged instruments during treatment.
2. Not forcing instruments.
3. Using instruments in the correct sequence, alternating sizes and tapers as appropriate.
4. Not rotating stainless steel instruments more than a quarter turn clockwise.
5. Confirming a glide path to size 20 with hand files prior to using rotary NiTi instruments.
6. Taking care with certain canal anatomy when using nickel titanium, e.g. canals that merge, divide or are dilacerated.
7. Ensuring straight line access before preparing the canals, thereby reducing stress on the instruments.

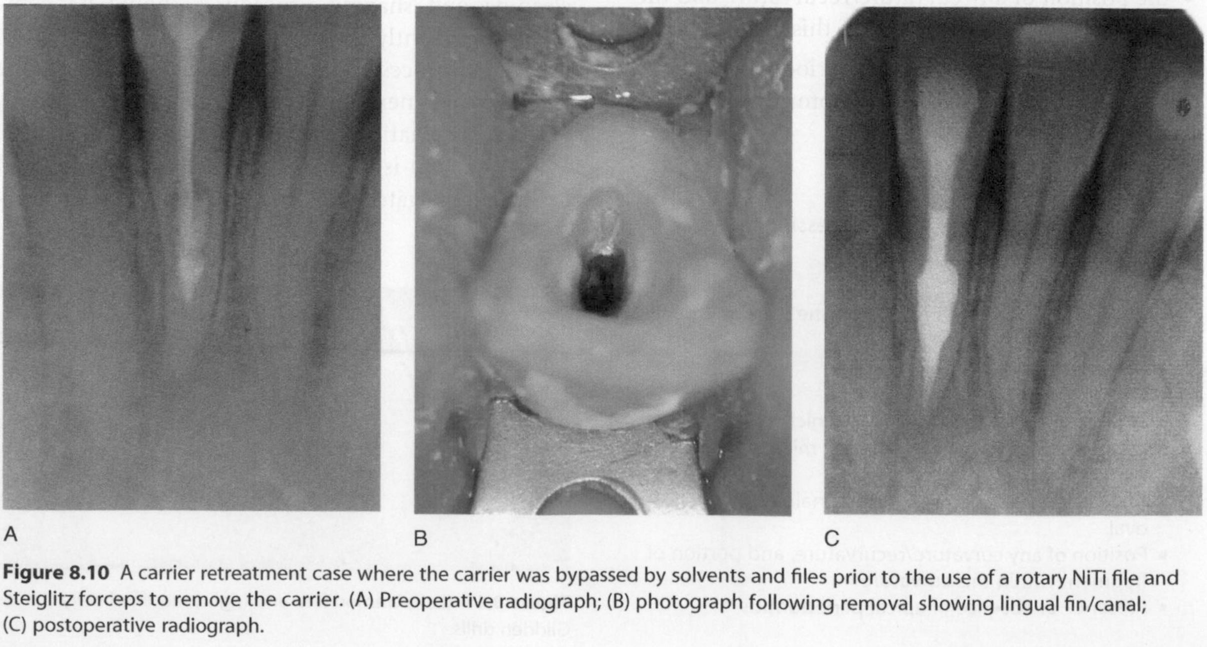

A B C

Figure 8.10 A carrier retreatment case where the carrier was bypassed by solvents and files prior to the use of a rotary NiTi file and Steiglitz forceps to remove the carrier. (A) Preoperative radiograph; (B) photograph following removal showing lingual fin/canal; (C) postoperative radiograph.

such as interfering with complete cleaning and disinfection of the canal. If the instrument has broken at length after thorough cleaning then it may be preferable to leave the instrument in situ rather than risk removing excessive amounts of tooth structure or perforating the root in a vain attempt at removal. It is also pertinent to put things into context as to the effect this unfortunate incident will have on the outcome of treatment. For example, if the instrument broke near the end of canal preparation in an uninfected case, then it is unlikely to affect the outcome. On the other hand, instruments that fracture early in the preparation of infected root canals will prevent thorough debridement and are therefore more likely to be associated with problems.

A thorough evaluation of the root containing a fractured instrument should be undertaken, including multiple radiographic angles (Box 8.5). Key information includes:

- the width and length of the fragment and whether it is stainless steel or nickel titanium — nickel titanium is more brittle than stainless steel and may fracture on contact with ultrasound
- location of the instrument — coronal, middle or apical third of the root
- the anatomical cross-section of the canal — round or oval
- the position of any curvature/recurvature and the portion of the fragment within this curvature
- presence or absence of apical periodontitis, either radiographically or clinical symptoms.

Box 8.5 Key considerations in assessing fractured instruments

- When the instrument broke — at the start or end of preparation
- Multiple radiographic angles
- Width and length of the fragment
- Type of metal — stainless steel or nickel titanium
- Location of instrument — coronal, middle or apical third
- Anatomical cross-section of the canal — round or oval
- Position of any curvature/recurvature, and portion of fragment within this curvature
- Presence or absence of apical periodontitis

Consideration of the above factors will influence choice of approach: orthograde, surgery or monitoring of the situation. Normally an orthograde approach would be considered the method of choice for easily accessible instruments in the straight part of the canal. Discretion is advised as one moves further apically, especially in curvatures, as removal attempts of more deeply placed instruments may weaken or perforate the root. In such situations surgery should be considered if treatment is required.

Stages in fractured instrument removal

These stages are firstly to improve radicular access and secondly to ensure good visibility to obtain a clear view of the instrument, using Gates-Gliddens and modified belly Gates-Gliddens (Fig. 8.11). The use of these instruments creates debris, and copious irrigation using NaOCl, EDTA and alcohol is required to help improve vision after drying and to assess the position of the instrument. Bypass should be attempted in the first instance, prior to attempting removal, as this gives an early indication of the anatomy of the canal. Care must be taken not to force instruments, however, as the broken fragment may direct the 'bypassing' file off line, with the danger of perforation. Bypassing instruments becomes more difficult in the apical third, as canals are normally rounder in cross-section in this area. If it is possible to bypass the instrument, then cleaning and shaping procedures should be completed. Frequently the instrument will be removed as part of the process, especially if a small ultrasonic file can be placed next to the instrument to flush it out, using a combination of gentle vibration and irrigation. If the fragment is not removed then the canal should be shaped, irrigated and obturated to include the frac-

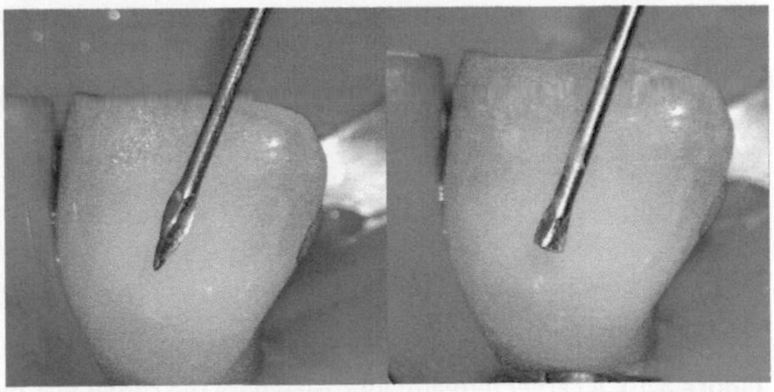

Figure 8.11 (Left) Unmodified and (right) modified belly Gates-Glidden drills.

tured instrument as part of the root filling, as in many situations success rate will not be affected.[5]

An operating microscope is required to aid visibility for removal of anything other than superficially placed instruments. Space may be created around the instrument using a small ultrasonic tip at low power, taking care to work in an anticlockwise manner around the fragment. This lateral trough should be continued to a depth of 2 mm, if possible, prior to applying vibration laterally against the instrument, which may then unscrew. Superficially placed fractured instruments may be grasped by a Masserann extractor or Ruddle IRS in a similar way to silver points (Fig. 8.12). Alternative removal methods include placing a small amount of chemically cured composite inside a spinal needle, or a small amount of superglue or composite inside a close-fitting Cancellier tube (Fig. 8.13), and placing the needle/tube over and around the exposed fractured instrument. The speed of set of the superglue can be accelerated by using a few drops of monomer, whilst the composite should be left for about 5 minutes before attempting manipulation of the fragment. Once set, the tube is rotated gently with an emphasis on anticlockwise movement in order to attempt delivery of the fractured instrument (Fig. 8.14).

Visibility decreases deeper in the canal, and in the case of an instrument that is completely placed in a curve, it may not be possible to see it at all. Ultrasound should be used at low power deep in the canal for dentine removal and file loosening. This will help avoid inadvertent dentine removal and disintegration

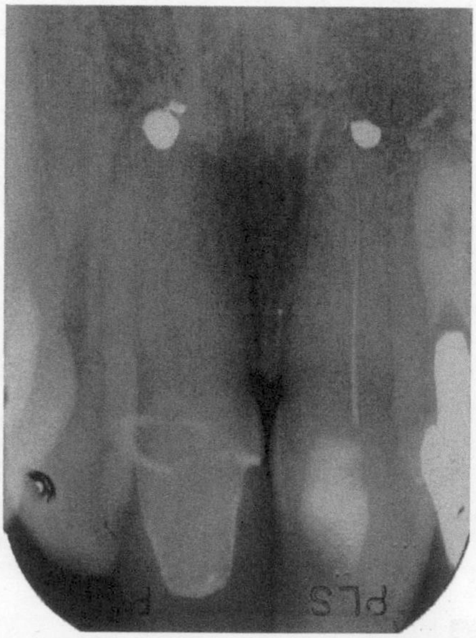

A

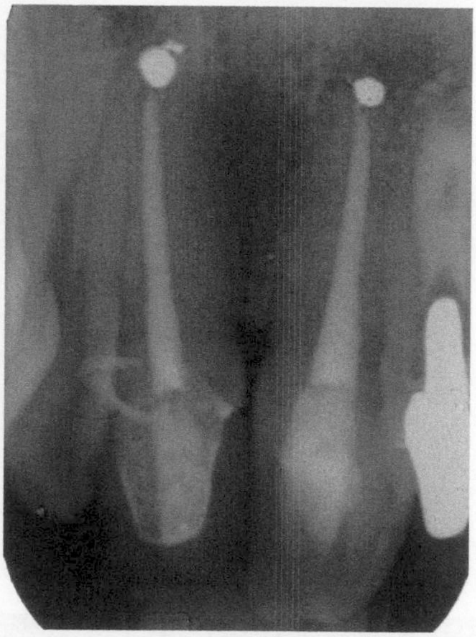
C

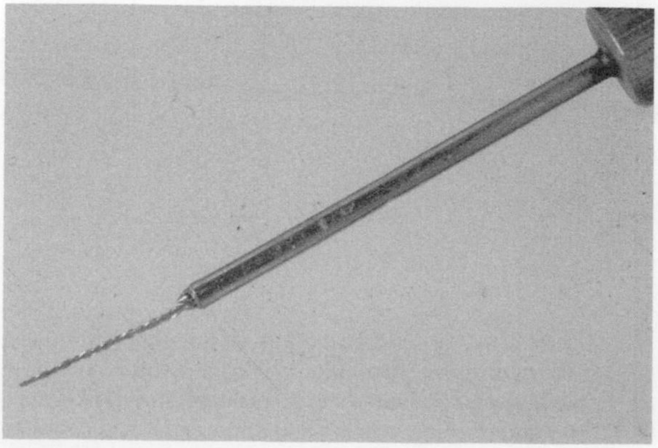
B

Figure 8.12 Superficially placed fractured instrument (A), removed with a Masserann extractor (B), following troughing (C).

of the only exposed part of an instrument that is slightly engaged in a curve. Delivery of the instrument may be complicated by it impacting against the outer canal wall as it is elevated, a situation that becomes more likely, the longer the instrument. In such situations space should be created laterally to allow the instrument to move in. File straightening can be especially problematic with NiTi fragments, as these straighten on release from curvatures, thereby continuing to lie tight against the canal wall and resisting attempts to place retrieval instruments around them. In such situations it may be possible to tease the fragment out with a series of precurved small stainless steel files, but this is unpredictable.

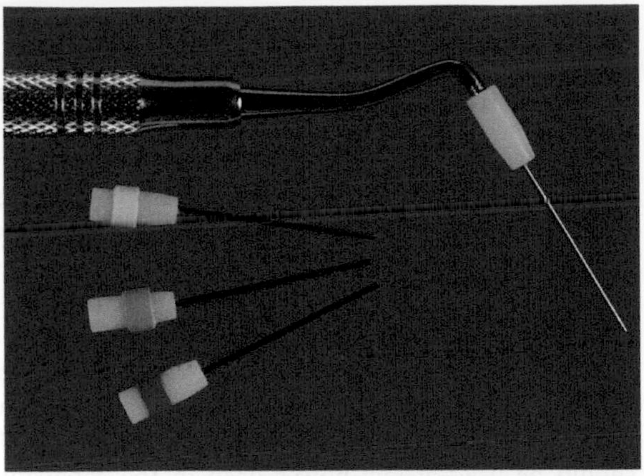

Figure 8.13 Cancellier tubes which may be used with superglue to help remove fractured instruments.

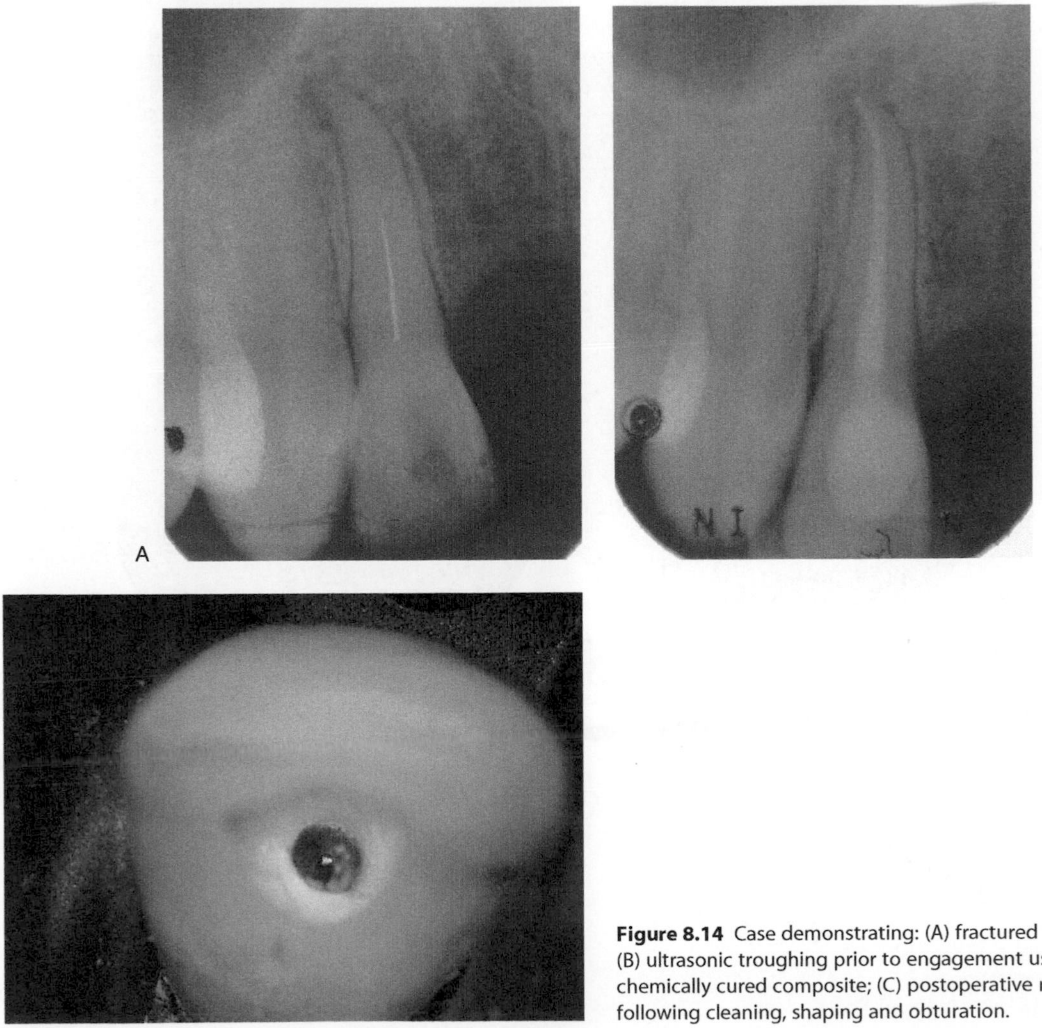

A

C

B

Figure 8.14 Case demonstrating: (A) fractured instrument; (B) ultrasonic troughing prior to engagement using tube and chemically cured composite; (C) postoperative radiograph following cleaning, shaping and obturation.

REGAINING CANAL PATENCY

Frequently, after removal of filling materials or broken instruments, blockage or a ledge will be noted, preventing further progress down the canal and completion of cleaning and shaping. The first stage is to refine the coronal and radicular access, as this creates space for thorough irrigation with NaOCl/EDTA, placement of a lubricant and introduction of a small file with a curve, placed in the apical few millimetres, using a file bender (Fig. 8.15). This instrument is directed towards the curvature and used to pick and probe the depths of the canal until a catch or bite is sensed. If this is not initially successful, then the file is removed and recurved or, alternatively, a new file substituted. Blockage and ledge negotiation may result in many small files being discarded. Once a bite is felt, then the file is moved in and out in small increments to smooth the path and advance apically. A very light watch-winding movement may also be employed with care. Files are advanced in this manner to the end of the canal, up to size 20, and the preparation may be smoothed using precurved 06 (white) and 08 (yellow) hand GT files in reverse balanced force, as described in Chapter 5.

PERFORATIONS

Perforations of the root canal may occur during root canal treatment. Breach of the pulp chamber floor in multi-rooted teeth during access, or labial perforation during access through crowned anterior teeth, are two of the more frequently encountered problems (Figs 8.16A,B and 8.17A,B), especially if there is limited visibility due to inflamed pulp tissue, or the canals are calcified. Several materials have been advocated for the management of perforations, with the current one of choice being mineral trioxide aggregate (MTA) in view of its tolerance of moisture and sealing ability. This material, however, requires a two-stage procedure and other single step techniques using barrier methods are still used occasionally.

The first stage of perforation management involves length determination using an apex locator and paper points, debriding/irrigating the area carefully to preclude a hypochlorite accident and then repair of the perforation. MTA is mixed to a stiff slurry, introduced to the site with a plastic instrument or suitable carrier (e.g. the Dovgan or Dentsply models) and tamped gently into place with a plugger. A damp pledget of cotton wool is then placed over the MTA, the access sealed, and the patient reappointed. At the next appointment the MTA is evaluated by dragging a probe over its surface to ensure its set, and the root canal is then obturated (Fig. 8.16C,D). If it is desired to complete all treatment in one visit, then a barrier, such as calcium sulphate (Calasept), may be placed in the periradicular tissues up to the root edge, and Super EBA or glass ionomer inserted, once moisture control is assured (Fig. 8.17C,D).

The success of perforation repairs is related to the length of time they have been present, degree of infection, and their size and relationship to the gingival margin. Perforations should be sealed as soon as possible, and the smaller they are the easier they are to deal with. Those closer to the cervical area are more likely to be associated with periodontal breakdown, whereas perforations in the apical third are frequently best managed surgically, as it may not be possible to renegotiate and obturate the apical few millimetres past the perforation.

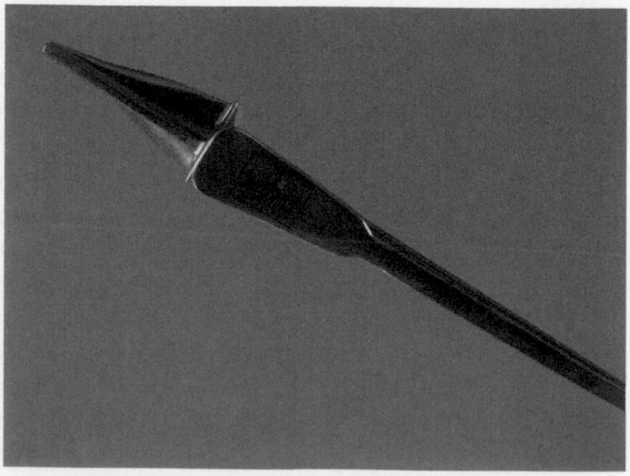

Figure 8.15 Buchanan file bender which may be used to place a small bend on the end of a file to help negotiate ledged canals.

ANTIMICROBIAL MANAGEMENT

Retreatment of teeth with apical periodontitis has a poorer prognosis than initial therapy, with infection at the time of treatment and the size of the lesion both influencing the outcome. Clinical ability to control infection in retreatment cases may be due to several factors:

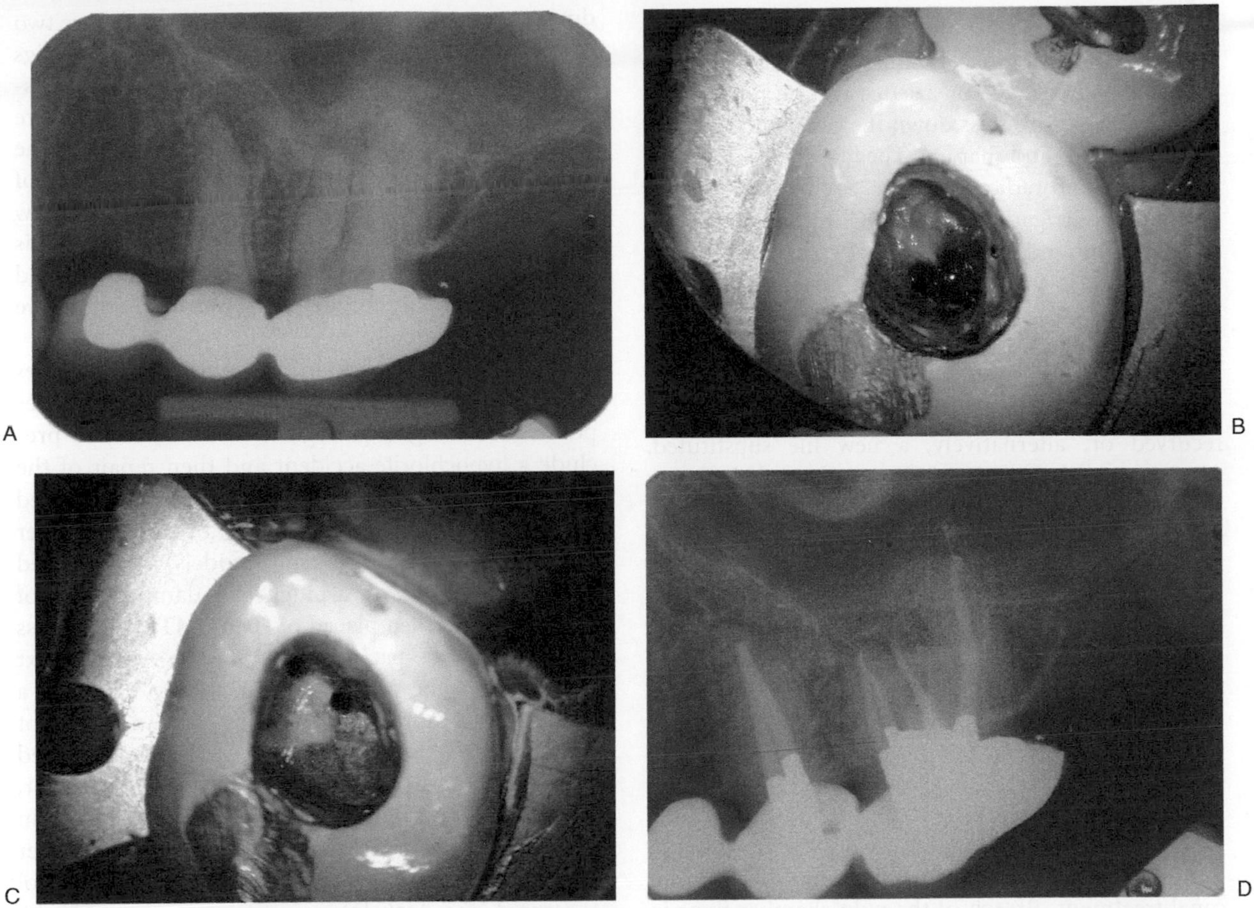

Figure 8.16 Furcal repair using grey MTA. (A) Preoperative radiograph; (B) perforation site; (C) MTA repair; (D) postoperative radiograph. No barrier was used in this case and although some furcal extrusion can be seen, this was uneventful.

- Bacteria lying in canal recesses may be protected by residues of filling material and thereby not exposed to antibacterial agents
- Existing ledges, transportation and obstructions may prevent an optimal level of debridement and root filling.

As stated earlier in this chapter, the aim of retreatment is to regain access to and treat infection within the root canal, the flora of which can be variable.[6] In cases where much of the root canal system has not been instrumented, then flora are likely to be polymicrobial in nature, similar to that of a necrotic pulp, and antimicrobial management follows conventional lines, i.e. thorough cleaning, disinfection and placement of calcium hydroxide ($Ca(OH)_2$). If the previous root treatment has managed most of the canal system, however, then the flora may be different, with only a few species being present. One organism that has been associated with such failures is *Enterococcus faecalis*,[7] which is resistant to elimination. Therefore, in such cases, a 10-minute soak with 5% iodine potassium iodide (IKI) following preparation and smear layer removal, has been advocated,[8] together with adding IKI to the usual $Ca(OH)_2$ intervisit dressing to help eradicate this organism. An alternative is to not use IKI but to add camphorated mono-chloro-phenol to a slurry of $Ca(OH)_2$ and glycerin as an intervisit root canal dressing.[9] Many operators prefer not to use IKI in view of its allergenic potential.

The success of root canal retreatment is good (94–98%)[10] when it is being undertaken to achieve a

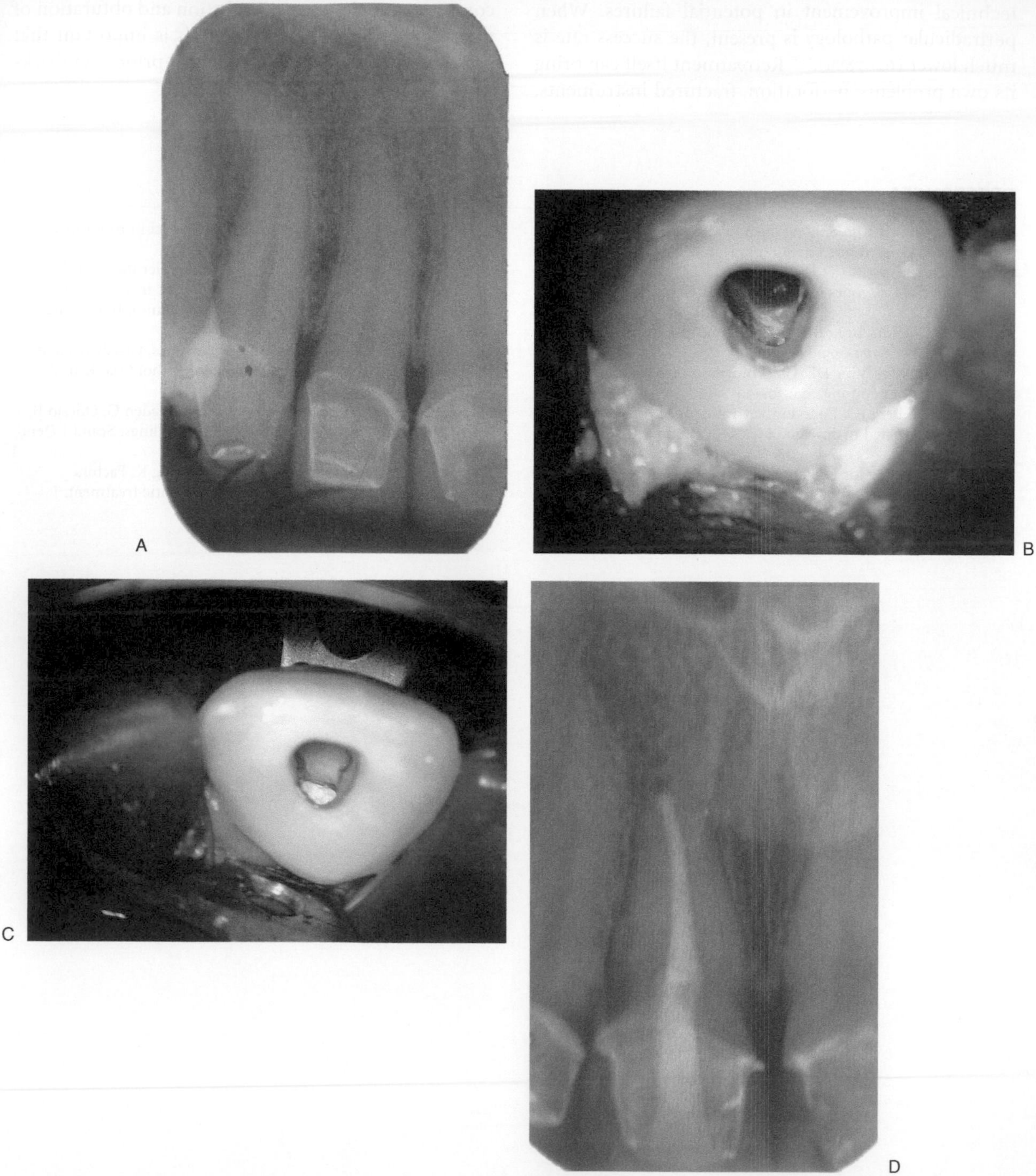

Figure 8.17 Labial perforation. (A) Preoperative radiograph; (B) labial perforation; (C) glass ionomer repair following placement of a barrier; (D) postoperative radiograph.

technical improvement in potential failures. When periradicular pathology is present, the success rate is much lower (62–78%).[10,11] Retreatment itself can bring its own problems: perforation, fractured instruments, compromised cleaning, disinfection and obturation of the root canal system. Therefore it is important that patients are informed of such factors prior to embarking on this procedure.

REFERENCES

1. Rubinstein RA, Kim S. Long term follow up of cases considered healed one year after apical microsurgery. J Endod 2002; 28: 378–383.
2. Carr GB. Microscopes in endodontics. J Calif Dent Assoc 1992; 20: 55–61.
3. Ruddle CJ. Non surgical endodontic retreatment. J Calif Dent Assoc 1997; 25: 769–799.
4. McDonald MN, Vine DE. Chloroform in the endodontic operatory. J Endod 1992; 18: 301–303.
5. Fors UGH, Berg JO. Endodontic treatment of root canals obstructed by foreign objects. Int Endod J 1986; 19: 2–10.
6. Sundqvist G, Figdor D, Persson S, Sjogren U. Microbiologic analysis of teeth with failed endodontic treatment and the outcome of conservative retreatment. Oral Surg 1998; 85: 86–93.
7. Engstrom B. The significance of enterococci in root canal treatment. Odontol Revy 1964; 15: 87–106.
8. Kvist T, Molander A, Dahlen G, Reit C. Microbiological evaluation of one and two visit endodontic treatment of teeth with apical periodontitis: a randomized clinical trial. J Endod 2004; 30: 572–576.
9. Siqueira JF. Endodontic infections concepts, paradigms and perspectives. Oral Surg Oral Med Oral Pathol Oral Radiol Endod 2002; 94: 281–293.
10. Bergenholtz G, Lekholm U, Milthorn R, Heden G, Odesjo B, Engstrom B. Retreatment of endodontic fillings. Scand J Dent Res 1979; 87: 217–223.
11. Sjogren U, Hagglund B, Sundqvist G, Wing K. Factors affecting the long-term results of endodontic treatment. J Endod 1990; 16: 498–504.

9 Periradicular surgery

Endodontic surgery has advanced enormously in recent years. An increasing understanding of the biological rationale for treatment, the use of microsurgical techniques and the development of new materials has revolutionized surgical endodontic practice. Surgeons within the dental profession have always viewed it with scepticism due to its poor success rate and its perceived difficulty. Historically it has been performed following unsuccessful primary treatment, regrettably without due care and attention being paid to the original treatment. Traditional endodontic surgery has many limitations, with five of the most common errors being described by Carr and Bentkover:[1]

- performing surgery on incompletely debrided or poorly obturated root canal systems
- failure to completely resect through the root
- failure to detect additional canals
- placement of extreme bevels
- failure to place the root end preparation in the long axis of the root.

The armamentarium now available to perform endodontic surgery has made it a precise and predictable treatment modality. The use of the microscope and microsurgical techniques have allowed more favourable outcomes, with Rubinstein and Kim[2] reporting up to 96.8% clinical and radiographic success after 1 year, and 91.5% after 5–7 years.

Microsurgery allows easier identification of the root apex and root canal anatomy. As a result, smaller osteotomies and shallower root resection angles can be achieved. With the use of the microscope and highly specialized instruments, a surgical environment for precise and predictable treatment can be produced, whereby 'blind assumptions', as in conventional endodontic surgery, are no longer necessary (Table 9.1).

EMERGENCY SURGERY — INCISION AND DRAINAGE

Drainage should be established in cases of acute infection, rather than relying on antibiotics, thus following the age-old principle, 'Never let the sun set on undrained pus'. Drainage can be established in different ways and is normally gained through the root canal. If this is not successful then consideration should be given to incising any fluctuant swelling. The objective of the incision is to drain any pus or exudates from within the tissues (Fig. 9.1). Care needs to be taken with the choice of anaesthesia. Options include:

- a nerve block away from the site of infection
- infiltrating locally with anaesthetic around, but not into, the swelling
- spraying ethyl chloride onto the site of incision.

If there is any doubt as to the nature of the swelling, or a sample is required for microbiological testing, then consideration should be given to aspirating the lesion with a wide bore needle and syringe prior to incision. The incision should be made in a swift, deliberate manner into the most fluctuant part of the swelling. The tip of the blade is used to puncture the mucosa and submucosa, then the incision is lengthened with a lifting action, so as not to put pressure onto the base of the swelling and potentiate the spread of the infection.

PERIRADICULAR SURGERY

Periradicular surgery is being performed less frequently than in the past; however, this may change due to the increase in placement of non-metallic post systems, and their subsequent difficulty in removal, if they should fail. Periradicular surgery includes apicectomy, retrograde filling, correction of iatrogenic errors, management of root fractures, root resorption, hemisection, root amputation, replantation and

Table 9.1 Comparison of conventional and microsurgical techniques

Procedure	Conventional surgery	Microsurgery
Identification of the apex	Difficult	Precise
Osteotomy	Large (10 mm)	Small (<5 mm)
Root surface inspection	None	Always
Bevel angle	Large (45°)	Small (<10°)
Isthmus identification	Nearly impossible	Easy
Retropreparation	Approximate	Precise
Root end filling	Imprecise	Precise

Based on Kim et al.[3]

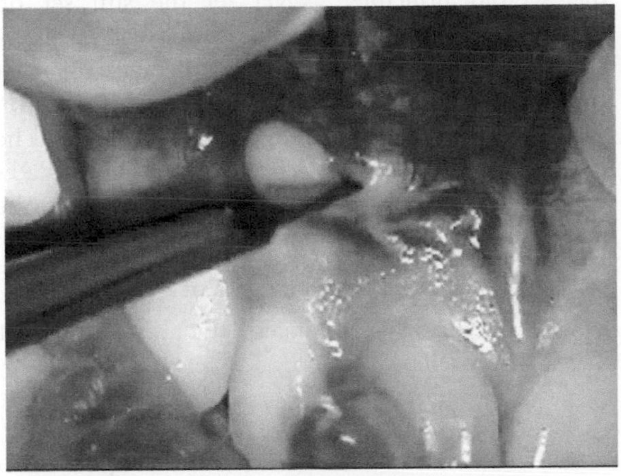

Figure 9.1 Surgical drainage of fluctuant abscess.

transplantation. A distinction should not be made between periradicular surgery and apical surgery in terms of their classification, as the term periradicular surgery encompasses all forms of surgery to the outer surface of the root.

Although there is an abundance of documented indications for surgery, conventional orthograde root canal treatment should be preferred,[4] even if it is considered that surgery still may be necessary at some time in the future. Such an approach reduces the bacterial flora within the canal system. If surgery is subsequently required there will be an increased chance of a successful outcome.

The most common indication for periradicular surgery is when persistent periapical infection exists, following technically good preparation and obturation of the root canal system after all orthograde approaches have been exhausted. Sometimes, following iatrogenic errors such as extruded filling material, root perforation and separation of irretrievable instruments within the root canal (Figs 9.2 and 9.3), surgery is often the only remaining treatment option. Frequently, tortuous roots do not permit complete debridement and obturation of the root canal system by conventional techniques, and in this instance surgery should be considered. On many occasions a definitive diagnosis cannot be made even following thorough assessment and direct visualization of the root surface — in such cases, biopsy may be required. In certain cases, patients are unwilling to have disassembly of expensive crown and bridgework for orthograde treatment of an endodontic problem, and surgery is the only alternative. A summary of common indications for periradicular surgery is presented in Box 9.1.

ASSESSMENT

It is important that a thorough assessment is made prior to embarking on surgery. General factors include the patient's medical history, in particular any factor that may contribute to problems with haemostasis and postoperative healing. Good haemostasis is crucial for visibility and moisture control. Conditions such as severe diabetes mellitus, neutropenia and leukaemia contraindicate surgery; however, the decision for treatment with any medical condition should be made on a case-by-case basis and liaisons with appropriate health care professionals should be sought.

Patient cooperation and suitability for a potentially lengthy procedure must be ascertained as part of the initial assessment. If the patient is anxious, conscious

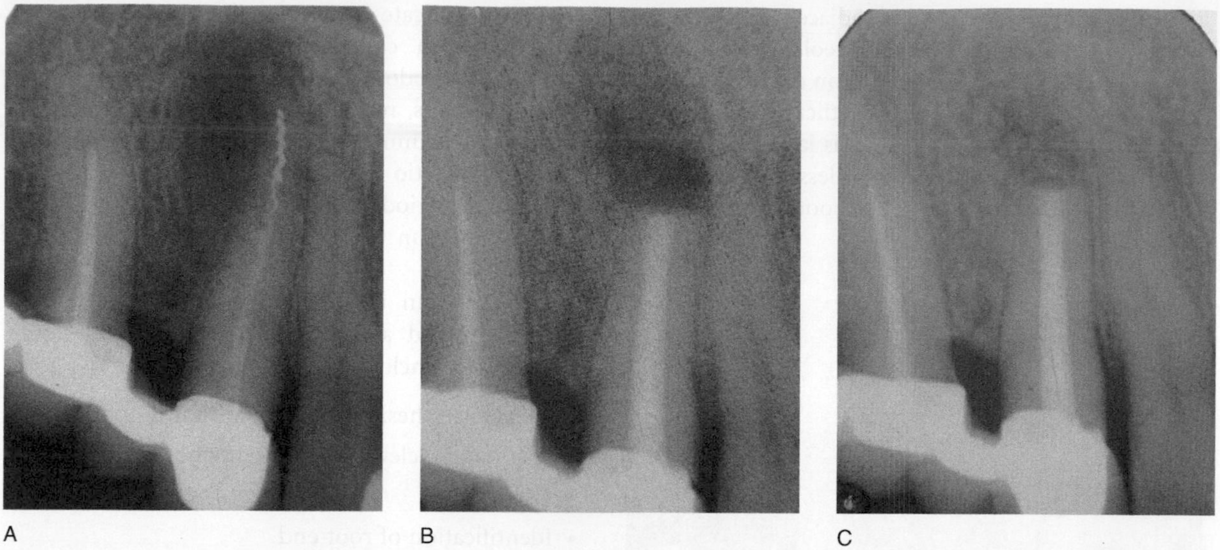

Figure 9.2 (A) Preoperative radiograph of periapical pathology associated with UR3 with retained instrument. (B) Immediate postoperative radiograph following apicectomy and root end filling with MTA after attempt at orthograde instrument retrieval. (C) 6 Month review.

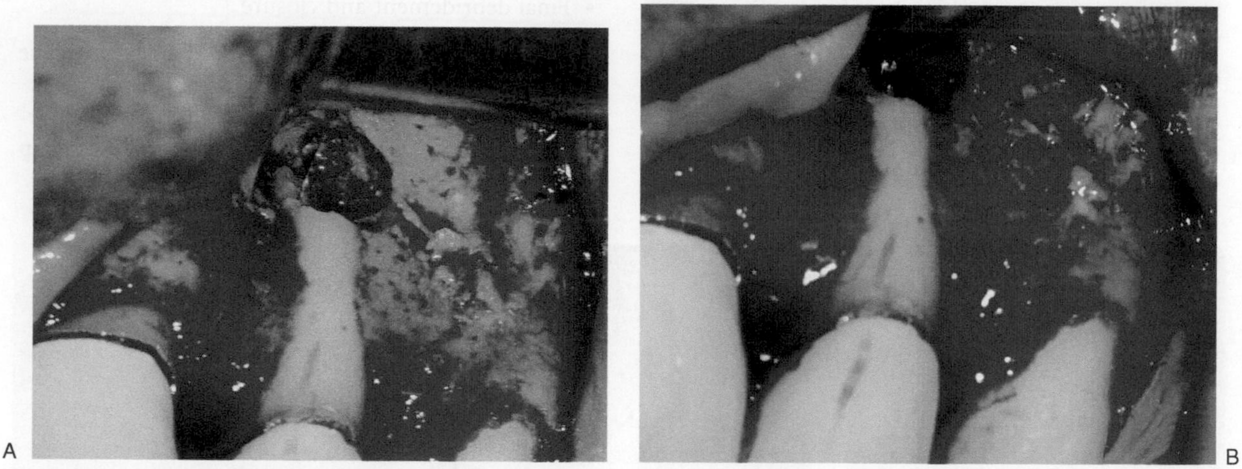

Figure 9.3 (A) Upper left lateral incisor with retained file present in canal. (B) File removal with fine needle holders. (Case courtesy of Mr G Bateman).

Box 9.1 Summary of common indications for periradicular surgery

- Persistent periapical infection following technically good orthograde treatment
- Iatrogenic errors
- Complex root anatomy
- Investigative surgery
- Unwillingness for disassembly of restorations

sedation should not be ruled out as an adjunctive therapy. Local factors include access to the periradicular tissues (in particular the resilience of oral tissues), sulcus depth, position of muscle attachments, tooth angulation and bone thickness (Fig. 9.4). Root end proximity to anatomical structures such as the maxillary sinus, mental foramen or inferior dental canal can be evaluated from angled radiographs. These will also give information on anatomical variations, such as

root curvatures, closeness of adjacent roots, extra canals and density/thickness of alveolar bone. Careful note should be made of the location of the pathology with regard to the root, i.e. whether it is lateral or apical (Fig. 9.5). If the pathology is lateral, then such cases should be re-root treated unless the resection is going to include that area of the root. Lateral lesions may also indicate a perforated post or root crack, therefore such cases deserve special attention. A thorough periodontal assessment is essential, noting probing depths, mobility and any possible perio- or endodontal communications. Special consideration to crown:root ratio should be made with regard to remaining periodontal attachment levels, as root length reduction will reduce periodontal support of the tooth.

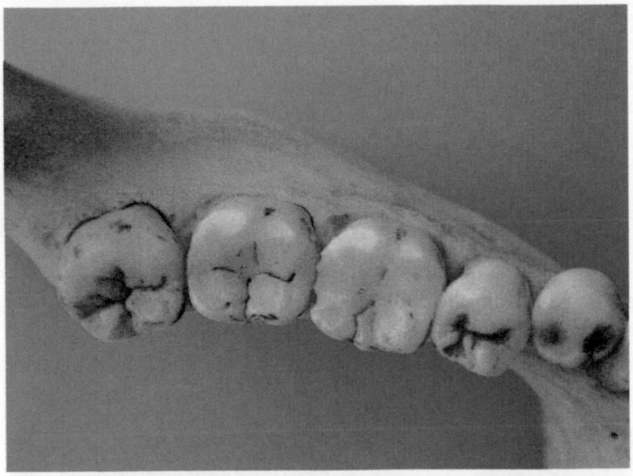

Figure 9.4 Thickness of the buccal cortical bone of left posterior mandibular teeth. Note: the thickness of buccal bone to be traversed before the root end would be reached in the second molar in comparison with the second premolar.

The case can be planned following appropriate assessment and a decision to perform endodontic surgery. This includes several distinct stages:

- Local anaesthesia and provision for haemostasis
- Flap design, elevation and retraction
- Osteotomy
- Identification of root end
- Periradicular curettage
- Root end resection
- Preparation and filling
- Final debridement and closure.

So that efficient use of time is made, the procedure should be considered in three phases (Box 9.2).

Prior to surgery, the patient should use a chlorhexidine mouth rinse twice in the 24 hours leading up

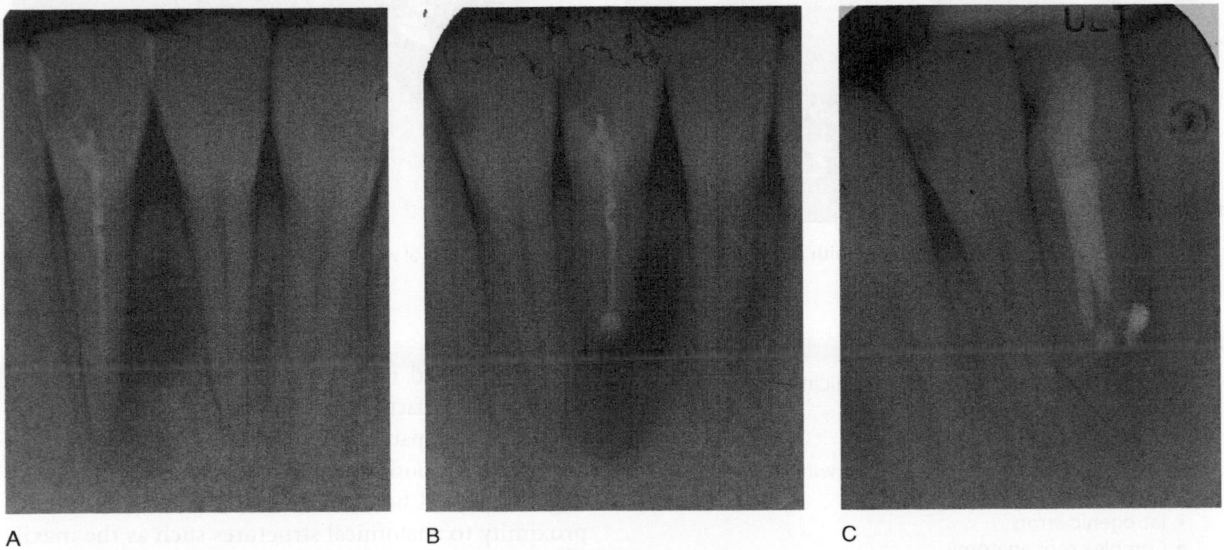

A B C

Figure 9.5 (A) Preoperative radiograph of a lower incisor with a large lateral lesion. (B) Apical surgery has been performed and failed due to lack of appreciation and attention to root canal anatomy. (C) Retreatment has been performed, demonstrating two canals and a large lateral canal. Healing has progressed but is not yet complete.

Box 9.2 The three phases of endodontic surgery

Phase 1	Local anaesthesia, flap design, incision and reflection
Phase 2	Osteotomy, curettage, crypt control, root end management
Phase 3	Radiograph, flap re-approximation, suturing, flap compression and postoperative instructions

to the surgery. This will reduce the bacterial load in the oral cavity and decrease the risk of a postoperative infection.[5] A suitable analgesic, such as paracetamol or ibuprofen, unless contraindicated, should be administered just before giving the local anaesthetic as this will reduce postoperative pain and discomfort.

Local anaesthesia

A topical anaesthetic ointment (e.g. benzocaine) should be left in place at the sites of injection for 1–2 minutes. Regional anaesthesia is administered as appropriate, followed by multiple local infiltrations around the apex of the tooth. Lidocaine HCL 2% and epinephrine are recommended. A concentration of 1:80 000 of epinephrine is used for regional anaesthesia; however, a concentration of 1:50 000 should be used locally around the surgical site, as this will aid haemostasis. Buckley et al[5] demonstrated that in bilateral posterior segment periodontal surgery, there was twice as much blood loss with patients that were anaesthetized with 1:100 000 epinephrine, compared to a concentration of 1:50 000.

Some 10–15 minutes should be allowed to elapse before the first incision is made, to allow adequate time for the anaesthetic solution to disperse into the tissues. Further attempts to improve anaesthesia or haemostasis once the flap has been elevated are often fraught with difficulty. It is important that none of the anaesthetic agent is deposited into skeletal muscle, as the epinephrine will stimulate B_2 adrenergic receptors, resulting in vasodilation. This will increase blood loss and a poor surgical field will develop. The anaesthetic solution should be deposited into numerous sites to ensure good distribution of the solution to the entire surgical area. It should be administered slowly (1–2 ml/min), as rapid injection causes pooling, resulting in delayed and limited diffusion into adjacent tissues.

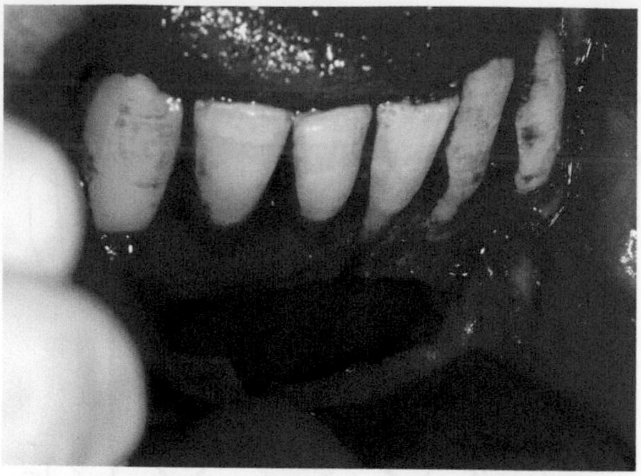

Figure 9.6 Reactive hyperaemia during lengthy surgery to remove periradicular cyst associated with all four lower incisors.

Lengthy surgery following administration of vasoconstrictor amines can result in a reactive hyperaemia or rebound phenomenon. When the local tissue concentration of vasoconstrictors no longer produces an alpha adrenergic effect, the restricted blood flow can rapidly increase to a flow rate well above normal (Fig. 9.6). This is due to a beta adrenergic effect resulting from localized tissue hypoxia and acidosis caused by the prolonged vasoconstriction. This can be reduced by immediate flap compression for 2–3 minutes following closure and the application of an ice pack to reduce tissue temperature and blood flow.

Flap design, elevation and retraction

Flap design

Atraumatic management of the soft tissue is an important part of surgery, as it decreases postoperative complications and maintains soft tissue aesthetics. The flap design should be planned prior to making any incision. A full thickness mucoperiosteal flap should always be performed for conventional endodontic surgery. Flap designs can be categorized into marginal flaps, submarginal flaps and hybrid flaps (Box 9.3) in terms of the shape of the flap and where the horizontal incision is made in relation to the gingival margin.

Marginal flaps In most cases, a marginal flap should be used, with either one relieving incision (triangular flap; Fig. 9.7A) or two relieving incisions (rectangular

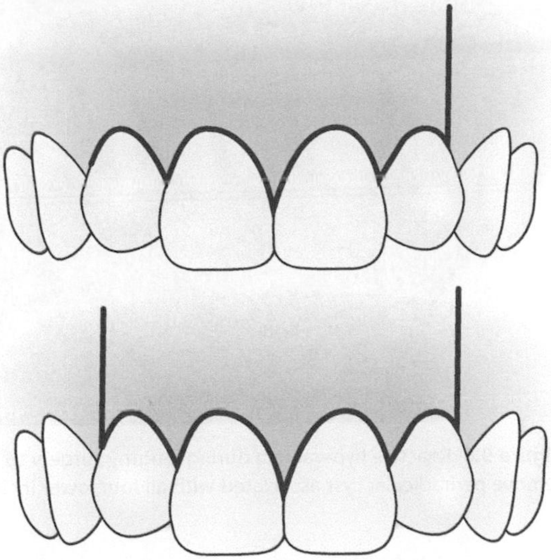

Figure 9.7 Flap design. (A) Marginal triangular flap; (B) marginal rectangular flap.

Box 9.3 Flap designs used in endodontic surgery

Marginal flaps
- Intrasulcular incision with one or two relieving incisions

Submarginal flaps
- Luebke Ochsenbein flap
- Semilunar flap
- Trapezoidal flap

Hybrid flap
- Papilla-based flap

flap; Fig. 9.7B). All relieving incisions should be made vertically and run parallel to the long axis of the tooth. As the vascular bed and fibre lines of the alveolar mucosa and gingivae run in this direction,[6] fewer blood vessels will be severed and the blood supply to the flap and non-flapped tissues is less likely to be compromised (Fig. 9.8). Care should be taken to avoid bony defects/dehiscence and root eminences. A distal relaxing incision may be used to relieve tension on triangular flaps to improve access. In the past, marginal flaps have been avoided, due to the risk of postoperative recession, especially if the aesthetics of indirect restorations could be compromised. Using the modern microsurgical techniques discussed in this chapter, this is rarely a problem.

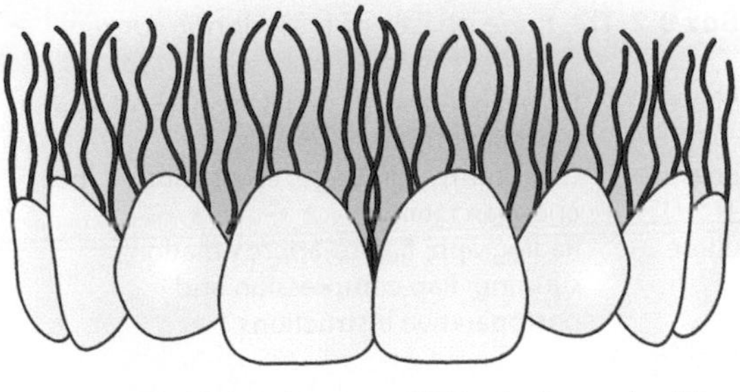

Figure 9.8 Blood vessels run parallel to the long axis of the teeth in the alveolar mucosa.

Submarginal flaps In cases where it is felt that a full marginal flap is not considered appropriate, then a limited submarginal flap can be used. The submarginal, semilunar and trapezoid flap should be avoided, as access is poor and scarring may result. These flap designs are of historic interest only due to scarring, inaccurate reapposition and limited access. The Luebke Ochsenbein flap is a horizontal scalloped incision with a 45° bevel that follows the gingival margin with two relieving incisions (Fig. 9.9). At least 2 mm of attached gingiva must remain apical to the depth of the gingival sulcus and there must be enough tissue to allow suture placement. Initial healing of submarginal flaps can be less predictable than marginal flaps; however, after 14 days there is no difference.[7]

Hybrid flaps Velvart[8] has recently introduced a new type of flap in surgical endodontics whereby the dental papilla is not raised as part of the flap, remaining attached to the palatal dental papilla by the midcol gingiva. It is suggested that, in patients with healthy periodontium, a papilla-based incision allows rapid, predictable and recession-free healing.

There are two flap designs for treating the palatal root of posterior maxillary teeth: an envelope intrasulcular flap design and a triangular flap. To achieve sufficient space in the envelope flap design, the incision and reflection of the mucosa should be made to the midline anteriorly (Fig. 9.10). If a relieving incision is employed this should be made between the canine and the first premolar. This is the junction at which the blood supply meets between the terminal branches of the sphenopalatine artery from the incisive canal anteriorly and the greater palatine artery posteriorly. A distal relaxing incision can be made along the maxillary tuberosity; however, when raising the flap

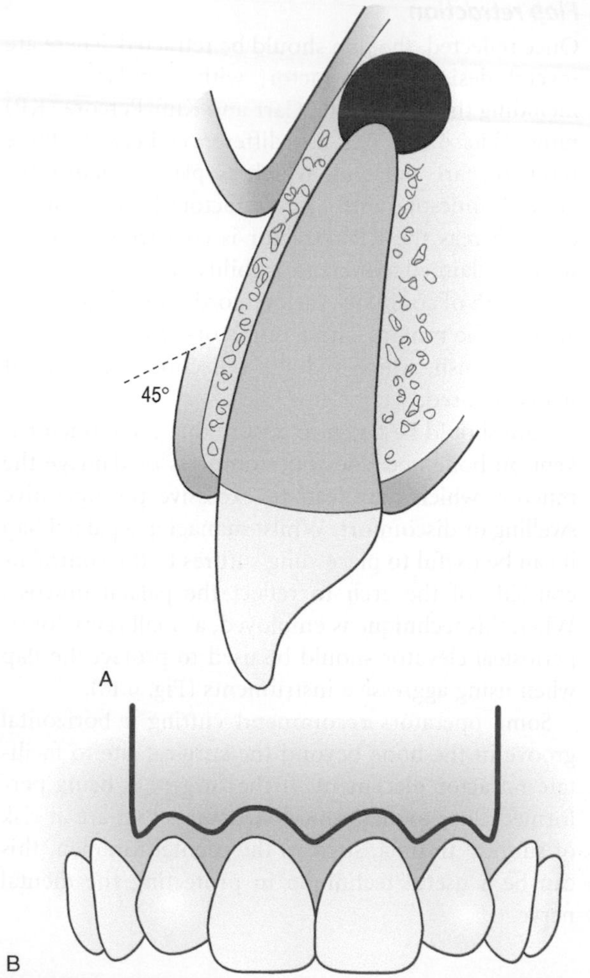

Figure 9.9 (A) Luebke Ochsenbein flap with vertical relieving incisions. (B) Cross-sectional view showing the 45° bevel for the horizontal incision.

great care should be taken in the region distal palatal to the second molar, where the greater palatine artery often emerges from its foramen.

Incisions for all flaps should be made with an appropriately designed scalpel blade, Nos 15 or 11 being frequently used. Recent developments, however, include the use of 15c or microsurgical blades (Fig. 9.11). The smaller microsurgical blades make it easier to dissect around the interdental papilla, especially in the midcol area separating the buccal and palatal papillae, thereby resulting in less trauma (Fig. 9.12).

Flap elevation

This should start at the attached gingiva on the vertical relieving incision. It then progresses laterally

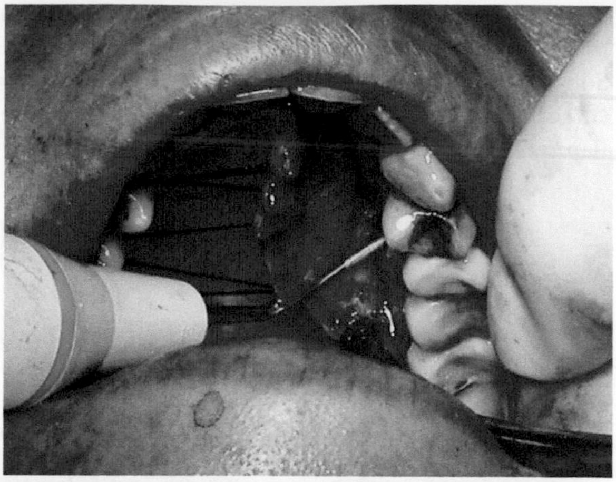

Figure 9.10 Reflected palatal flap with envelope design for access to the palatal root of the first molar. The flap is retained by silk sutures attached to the contralateral side of the arch; root end preparation is being carried out.

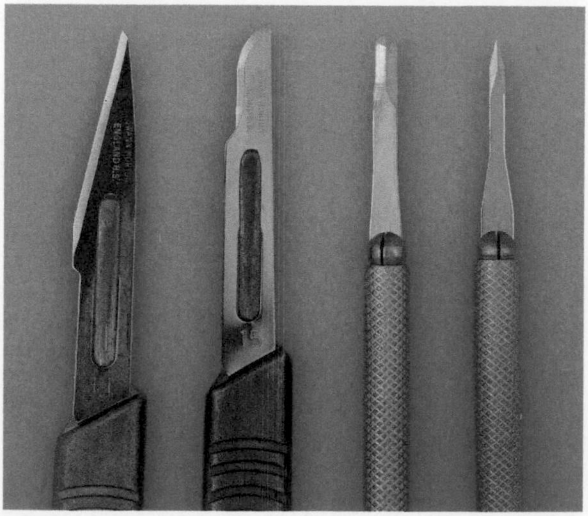

Figure 9.11 Conventional blades (Nos 11 and 15) with microsurgical blades.

(undermining elevation) to prevent damage to the flap margins associated with the cervical areas of the teeth. It is important to use sharp instruments to raise the flap as atraumatically as possible, as this will affect the quality of healing. Examples of suitable instruments include the Ruddle right and left and Molt curettes (Fig. 9.13). Care should be taken when lifting palatal mucosa as it is tightly bound to the bone and considerable force may be required to elevate it. Therefore, once the marginal areas of the flap are elevated, it is wise to use a large periosteal elevator as finer

instruments can sever and puncture the flap which may result in damage to the greater palatine artery. Soft tissue attachments, exostoses and previous surgery may all interfere with the clean raising of the flap.

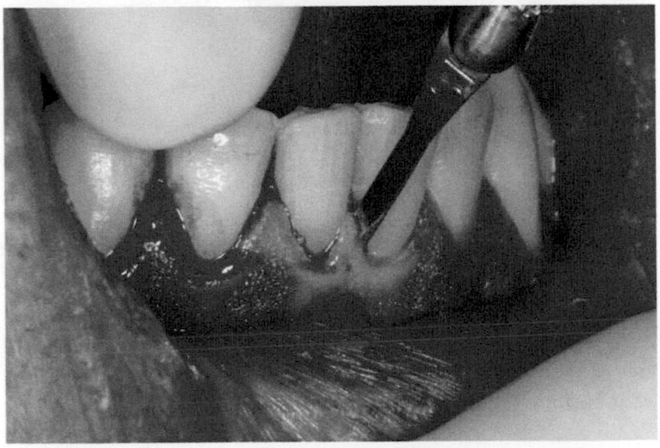

Figure 9.12 An SP 90 microsurgical blade predictably dissecting the midcol gingiva interproximally between the lower central incisors.

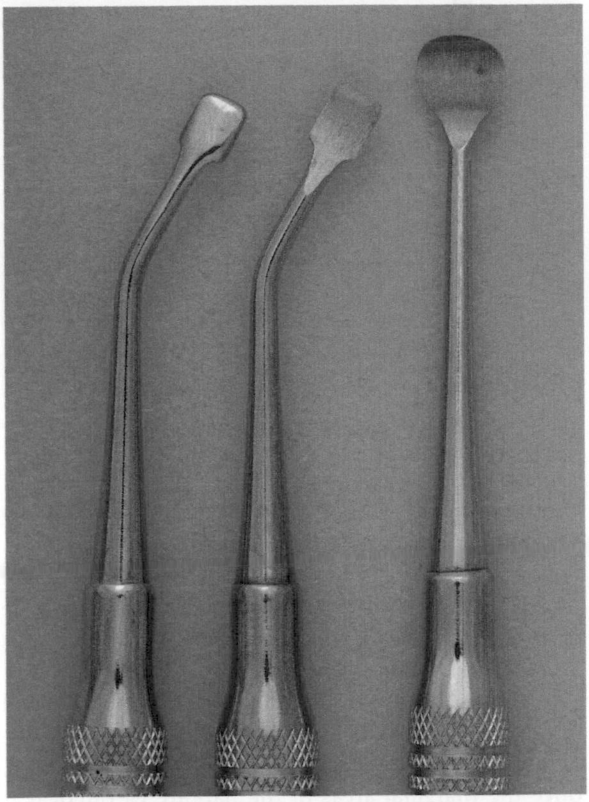

Figure 9.13 Ruddle right and left and Molt instruments.

Flap retraction

Once reflected, the flap should be retracted. There are several designs of retractor, with popular choices including the Minnesota, Carr and Kim-Percora (KP) range (Fig. 9.14). The key differences between these retractors are the end, which is placed against the bone. Minnesota and Carr retractors have a convex end, whereas the KP retractor is concave (Fig. 9.15), which is claimed to increase stability during retraction. The depth of concavity varies in order to suit different areas of the mouth. These retractors also have a matt surface finish, which reduces reflection when bright lights are used.

Care should be taken to ensure that the retractor is kept on bone and does not compress or damage the mucosa, which may lead to excessive postoperative swelling or discomfort. Whilst managing a palatal flap it can be useful to place sling sutures to the contralateral side of the arch to reflect the palatal mucosa. When this technique is employed, a small retractor or periosteal elevator should be used to protect the flap when using aggressive instruments (Fig. 9.16).

Some operators recommend cutting a horizontal groove in the bone beyond the surgical site to facilitate retractor placement. If the surgery is being performed close to anatomical structures that are at risk of surgical trauma, such as the mental foramen, this can be a useful technique in protecting the mental nerve.[3]

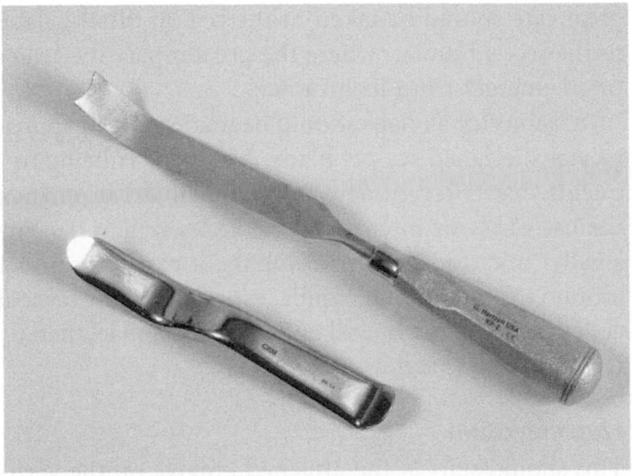

Figure 9.14 Minnesota and KP retractors.

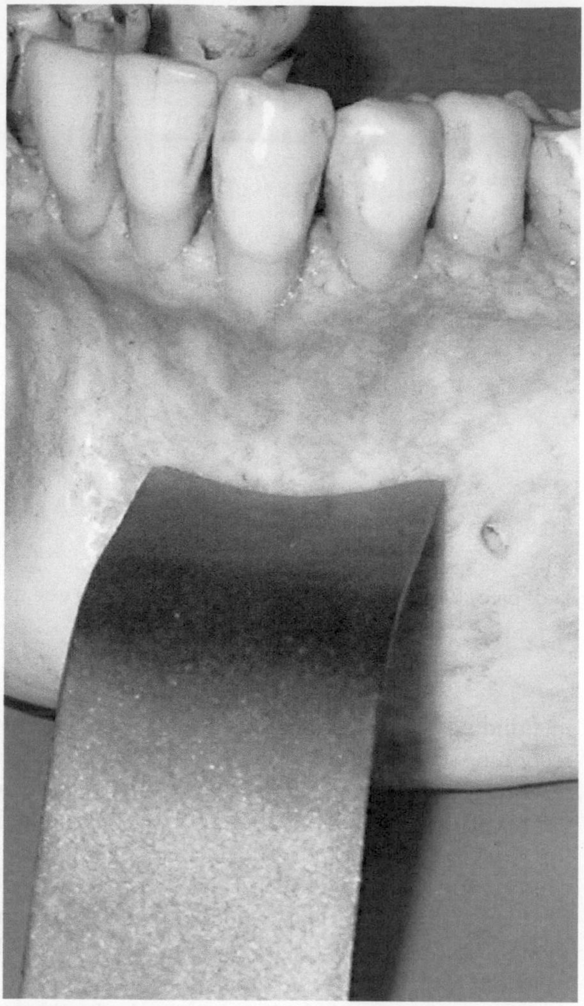

Figure 9.15 The concave KP retractor placed against the convex alveolus of a dry skull.

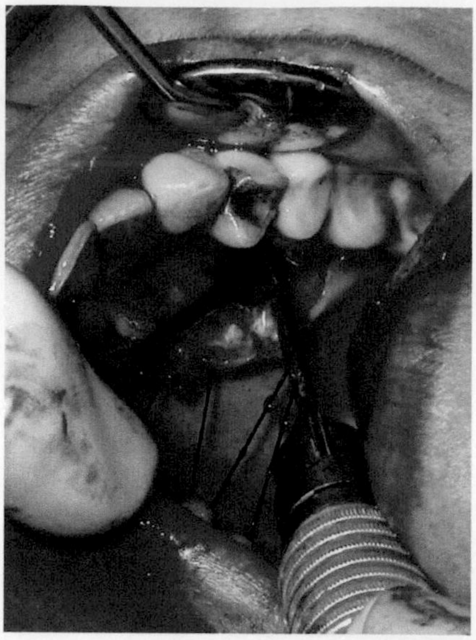

Figure 9.16 A periosteal elevator protecting the palatal mucosa during osteotomy with a straight handpiece.

Osteotomy

In most cases location of the root end is straightforward, especially if there is a large bony defect (Fig. 9.17). If there is a periapical radiolucency on radiographic examination, then the cortical plate is likely to be perforated or at least thinned[9] (Fig. 9.18). Therefore, the use of a DG16 is useful to explore the cortical plate and identify thin areas of bone. Following this, a round bur may be used to remove bone overlying the root and enable identification of the root apex. Care must be taken not to damage adjacent roots. The use of a dry skull is excellent to familiarize oneself with the topography of the alveolus and its relation to the root apex.

Good preoperative clinical and radiographic assessment will be reflected at this stage when trying to identify root apices. For instance, if splayed roots on upper premolars or very lingually inclined lower incisors are noted, then bone removal can be made with more confidence when trying to identify the root end. Operator preference will determine the type of handpiece used for bone removal and root resection, with many preferring the straight handpiece. However, suitable alternatives that give a greater degree of flexibility include the Impact Air 45° rear exhaust turbine (Fig. 9.19). This provides the increased efficiency of a high-speed handpiece without the risk of surgical emphysema. Popular burs for bone removal include the round No. 6 and the Lindeman bone bur. It is important to be definitive at this stage, as a bony access that is too small may not be conservative in the long run.

Bone removal may start at the junction of the apical and middle thirds of the root, with the bur being used in a side-to-side sweeping motion rather than aiming straight for the root apex. Ideally, the bony access should be the complete mesial to distal width of the root and a little bit more. To distinguish clearly between root dentine and bone, one should carefully observe colour and form. The root dentine will be darker, yellowish and hard, whereas bone will be soft,

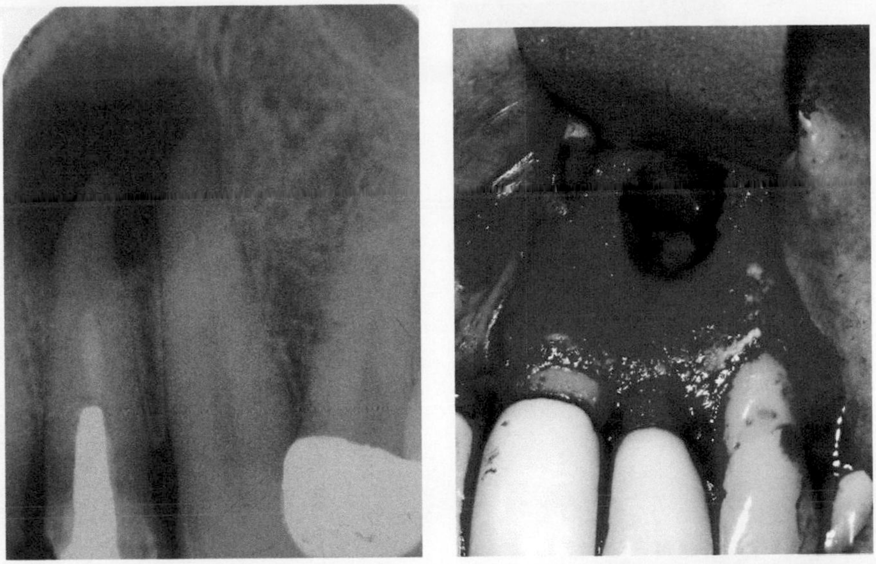

Figure 9.17 Large bony defect. (A) Preoperative radiograph showing large periapical area. (B) Partial debridement shows the extent of the bony lesion.

whiter and will bleed if scraped with a probe. Care should be taken to ensure sufficient crestal bone remains, at least 3 mm, but preferably 5 mm. The size of the osteotomy is primarily dependent on the size of the instruments used to prepare the root end. This will be discussed later in the chapter.

Once access to the root end has been achieved, it is necessary to curette out any soft tissue from the defect using curettes and jacquettes. A suitable sample of excavated tissue should be sent for histological examination. Haemostasis at this stage will not be at its optimum, as granulation/inflammatory tissue is highly vascular, and therefore further infiltration of local anaesthetic with a vasoconstrictor may be required. Histologically, the inflammatory tissue of the periradicular lesion is very similar to healing granulation tissue. Therefore if the lesion is close to an anatomical structure such as the mental nerve or maxillary antrum, it may be wise to leave this tissue as these structures could be compromised. As long as the root end or aetiological factor has been removed, normal healing will result.[10]

Root end resection

The root end may be resected using a fissure bur (170 plain cut tungsten carbide or a Lindeman bur), either by grinding it from an apical to coronal direction, or sectioning straight through. Care should be taken with the latter method, as more root may be removed than desired if the thickness of the bur is not accounted for. However, it may be preferred in anatomically compromised situations such as close to the mental foramen or the maxillary antrum. The resection should pass entirely through the root and care should be taken to avoid adjacent teeth.

In general, 3 mm of the root end should be removed,[11] as this should result in removal of the apical delta,[12] which may have been contributing to the failure of the case. Considerable debate exists as to the angle of bevel; ideally it should be 90° to the long axis of the root. This ensures that infected apical anatomy is removed while maintaining maximal root length (Fig. 9.20). Gilheany et al[13] found a positive correlation between increasing the bevel angle and apical leakage. Therefore no bevel is to be preferred. The 90° bevel will expose less dentinal tubule and thus reduce the portholes for leakage (Fig. 9.21). The advantages of zero bevel angle are summarized in Box 9.4.

At times, however, visibility can be problematic, and in such situations it may prove prudent to increase the angle of the bevel to simplify the procedure. This ensures that all canals and any isthmus have been identified and cleaned. To make certain that the com-

plete root end has been resected, methylene blue stain can be used to identify the whole of the periodontal ligament (Fig. 9.22).

Crypt control and haemostasis

Haemostasis is a critically important aspect of periradicular surgery, especially during root end inspection, preparing the retrograde cavity and placing the root end filling. Provisions for this stage have already been made when the local anaesthetic was administered. Now, further techniques and materials can be used to enhance the surgical field, as summarized in Box 9.5.

The choice of materials depends upon individual preference; however, any non-resorbable material placed in the surgical site should be counted on placement and removal to ensure that it is not left in situ on closure. Particular care should be taken with ferric sulphate, as it is a necrotizing agent and can cause tissue destruction, especially if placed on the cortical plate or soft tissue. It should only be used as a last resort and never near a neurovascular bundle or sinus membrane. Ferric sulphate may be applied in small

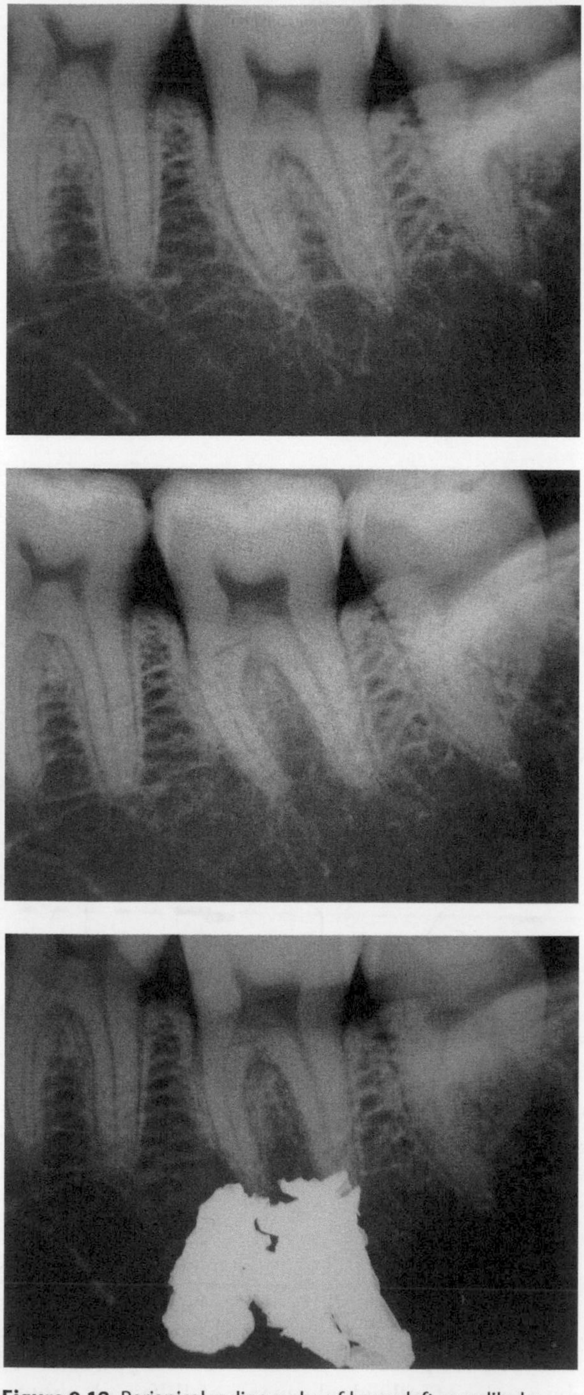
A
B
C

Figure 9.18 Periapical radiographs of lower left mandibular molars in dry skull. (A) Preoperative radiograph. (B) Second molar extracted and removal of periapical bone using slow-speed handpiece through the socket, therefore maintaining cortical plates. The tooth is then replaced (note the loss of lamina dura). (C) Insertion of lead foil to show extent of simulated periapical lesion.

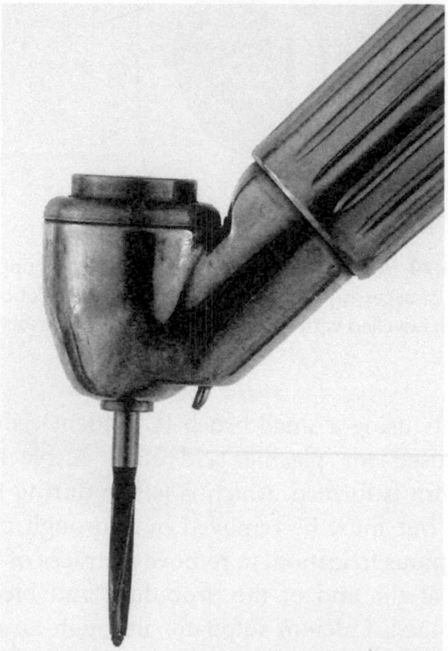

Figure 9.19 Impact Air 45° rear exhaust turbine with Lindeman bone bur.

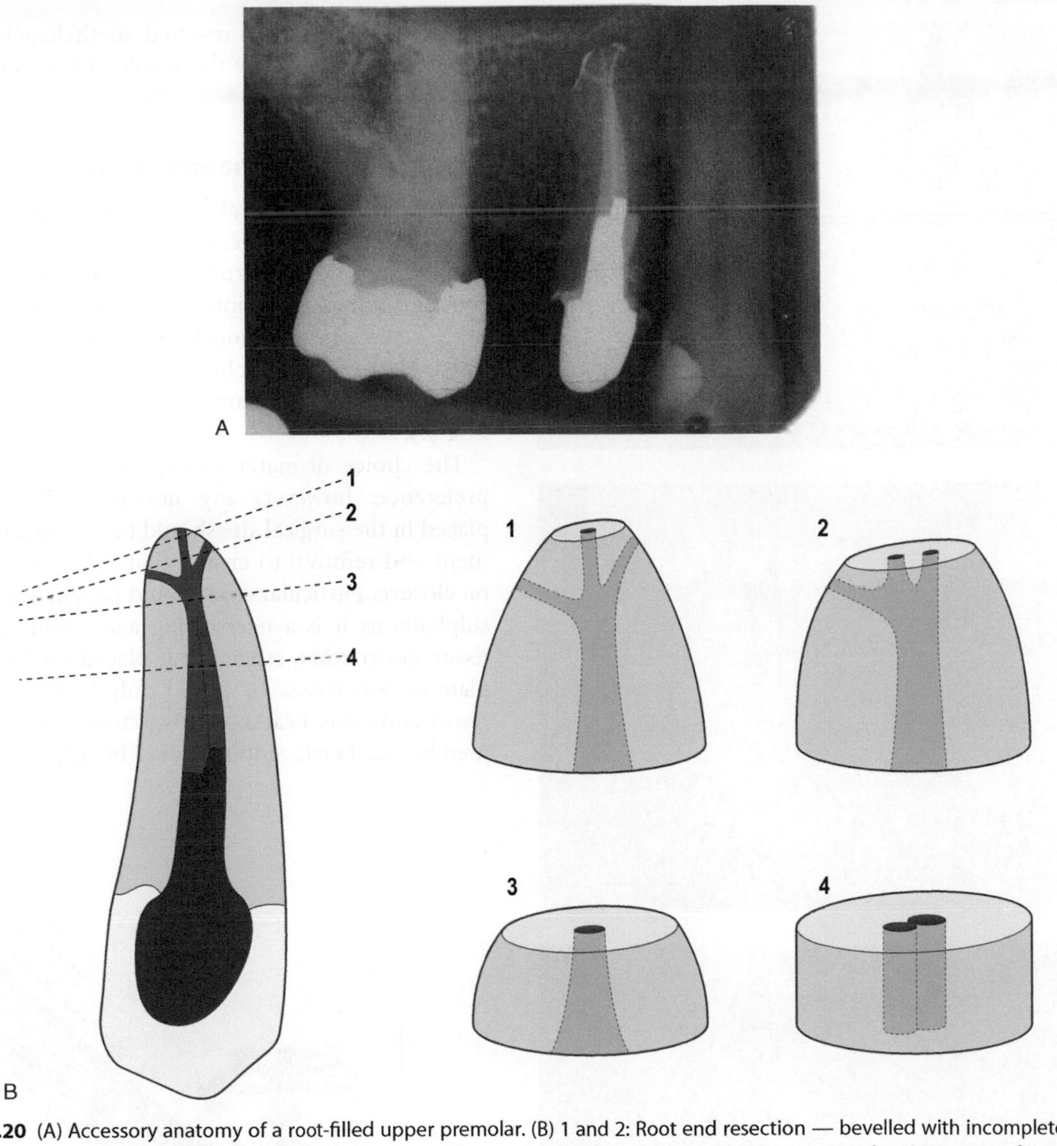

Figure 9.20 (A) Accessory anatomy of a root-filled upper premolar. (B) 1 and 2: Root end resection — bevelled with incomplete removal of accessory anatomy; 3: 90° root end resection with complete removal of accessory anatomy and maintenance of root length; 4: bevelled with complete removal of accessory anatomy but compromised root length.

amounts using a small brush (Ultradent), similar to those used for placing acid etch. A black/brown coagulum is formed, which is left in during the procedure but must be removed by thorough curettage and copious irrigation, to remove all traces of the substance at the end of the procedure and bleeding is encouraged. Calcium sulphate, although an effective haemostatic agent, is expensive and rarely used. The material is packed to excess and then carved back to expose the root end.

A popular current choice for haemostatic agents is the combination of epinephrine-containing pellets — Racellets (Fig. 9.23) — and Telfa pads. Two or three Racellets are placed in the base of the crypt, followed by a series of individual squares of Telfa pads about a centimetre in diameter, until the crypt is full (Fig. 9.24). Pressure is applied for a few minutes, prior to removing some of the Telfa pads and inspecting the root surface. The root end is examined using a microsurgical mirror, which is considerably smaller than a

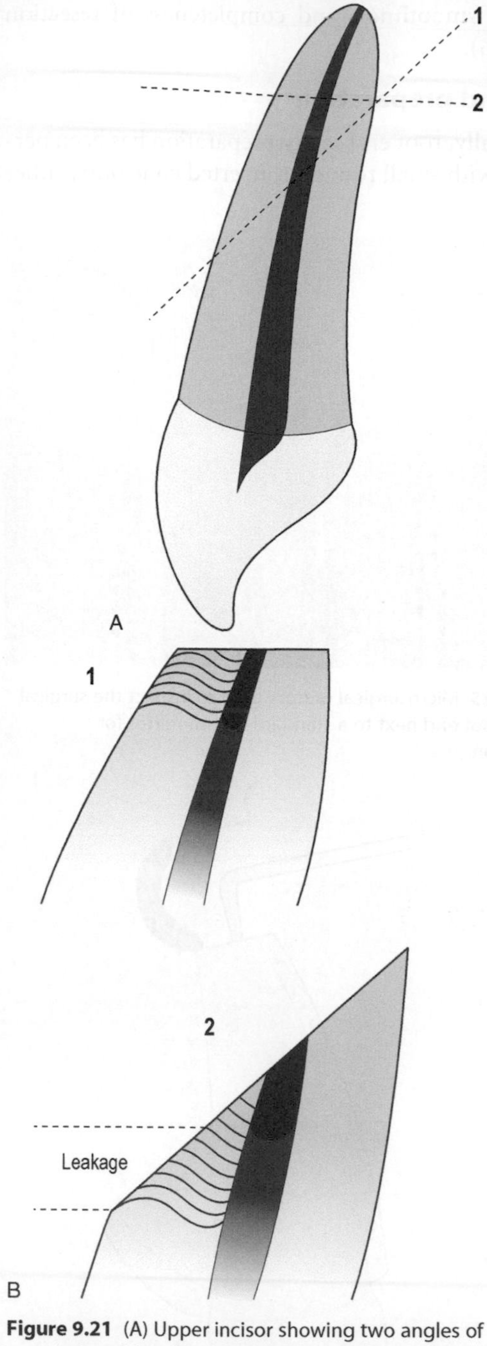

Figure 9.21 (A) Upper incisor showing two angles of resection — 1: reduced bevel; 2: excessive bevel. (B) A reduced bevel angle (1) exposes less dentinal tubule than an excessive one (2), which may result in less leakage.

Box 9.4 Advantages of a zero degree bevel

- Exposure of fewer dentinal tubules — decreased surface area of exposed root face
- Maintains maximum root length and still removes apical delta (Fig. 9.20B)
- Reduces osteotomy size

Box 9.5 Summary of haemostatic agents

Mechanical agents
- Bone wax

Chemical agents
- Ferric sulphate (Cut Trol)
- Epinephrine-impregnated cotton wool (Racellets)
- Collagen

Resorbable haemostatic agents
- Surgicel
- Calcium sulphate

Others
- Cautery

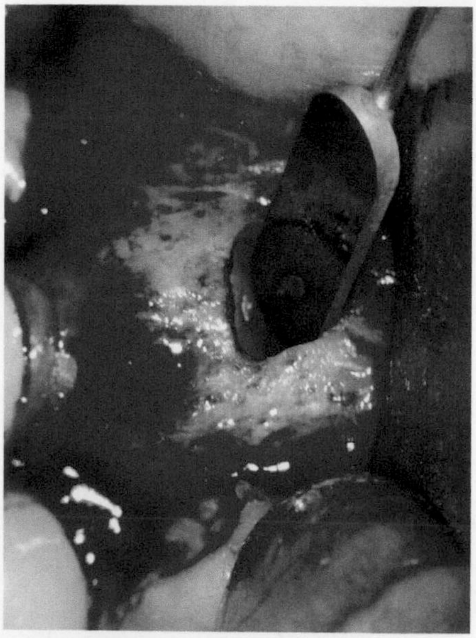

Figure 9.22 Methylene blue dye may be used to stain the periodontal ligament to ensure the root end is completely resected.

standard mouth mirror (Fig. 9.25) and small enough to fit into the surgical site to inspect the resected root end. These small mirrors have a tendency to steam up but this can be reduced by placing them in warm water. The root end should be examined using a microexplorer for cracks, unidentified canals, an isthmus, smoothness and completeness of resection (Fig. 9.26).

Root end preparation

Historically, root end cavity preparation has been performed with small round or inverted cone burs, either

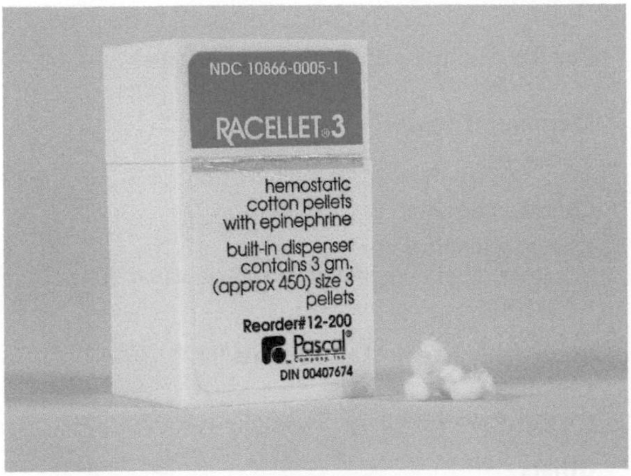

Figure 9.23 Cotton wool pellets impregnated with epinephrine to aid haemostasis.

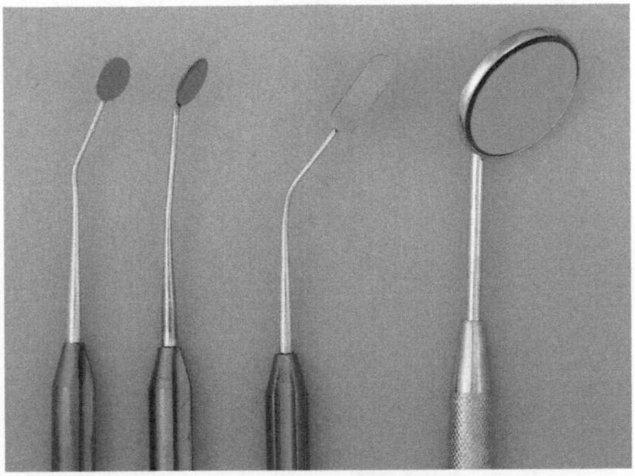

Figure 9.25 Microsurgical mirrors used to inspect the surgical site and root end next to a standard mouth mirror for comparison.

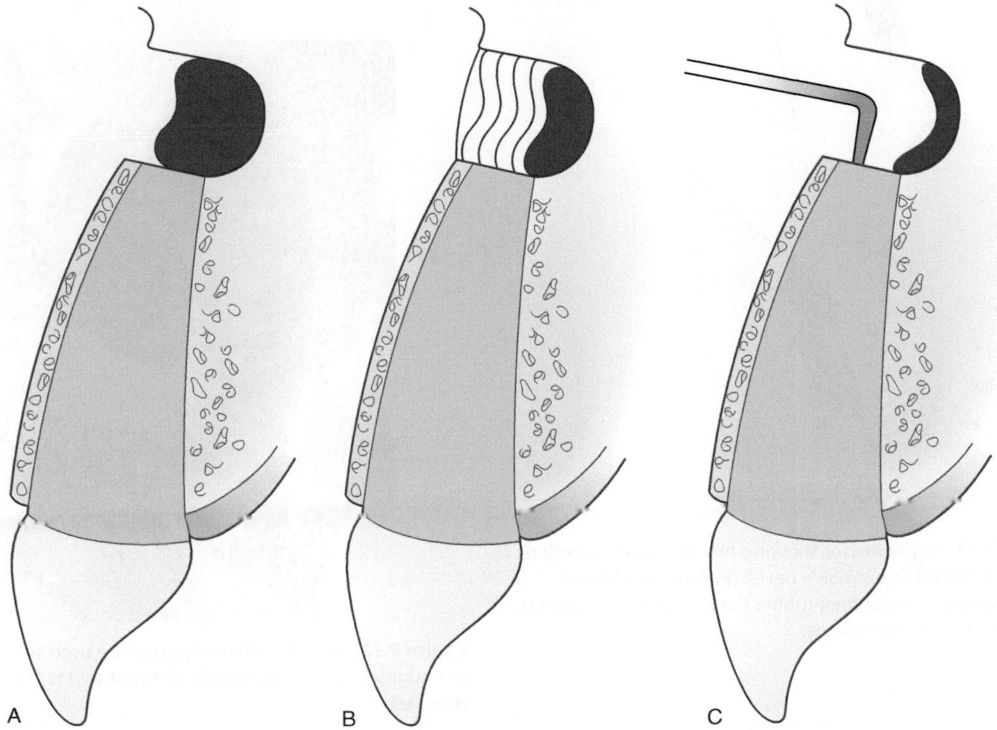

Figure 9.24 Bony crypt control. (A) Placement of two or three Racellets in base of crypt, followed by (B) Telfa pads and pressure with a blunt instrument for 2–3 minutes. (C) Removal of Telfa pads, but Racellets left in situ to collect any excess material at the root end filling stage.

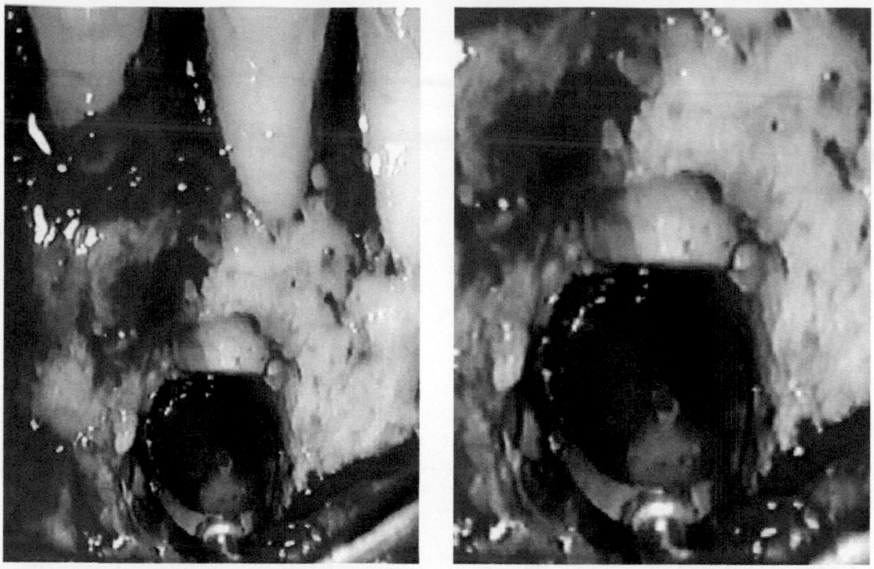

A B

Figure 9.26 (A) Low magnification view of lower incisor root end showing gutta-percha root filling and lingual fin. (B) Higher power view of canals.

A B

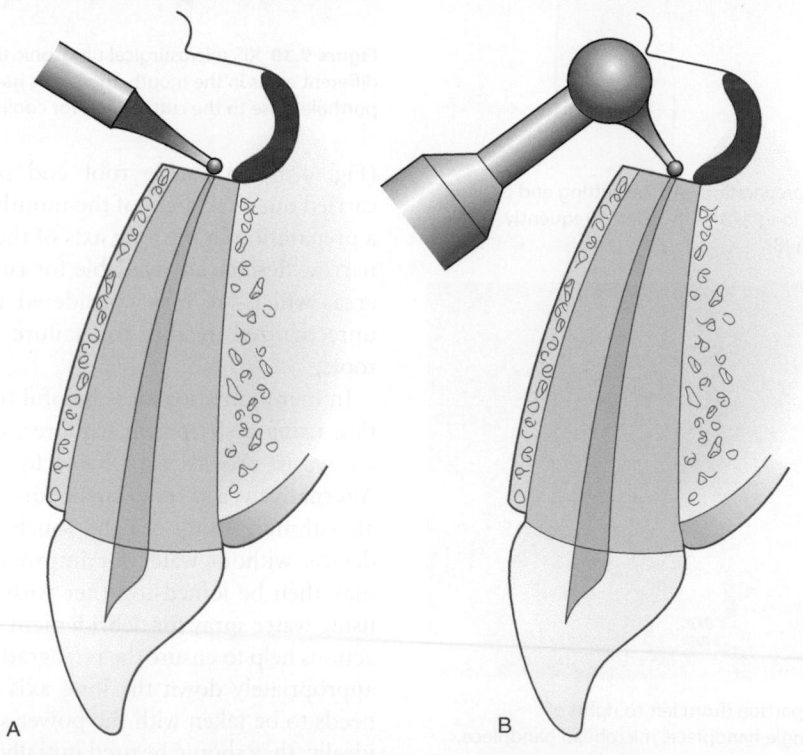

Figure 9.27 Root end preparation. (A) With straight handpiece; (B) with microhead handpiece.

in a straight or miniature handpiece (Fig. 9.27). It is difficult, however, even with a miniature head, to place the cavity preparation in the long axis of the root, in view of limited access. Frequently, although such preparations appear to be placed in the long axis of the tooth, they are in fact directed palatally, and occasionally with a palatal perforation (Fig. 9.28).

Recent developments have seen the introduction of ultrasonically activated microtips, which are much smaller than conventional instruments (Fig. 9.29),

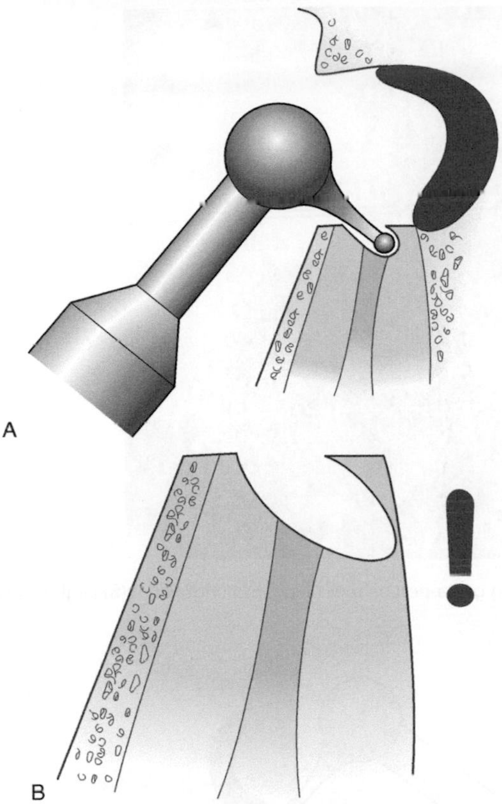

Figure 9.28 Bur retropreparation. (A) The cutting end is difficult to align in the long axis of the tooth, frequently resulting in perforation (B).

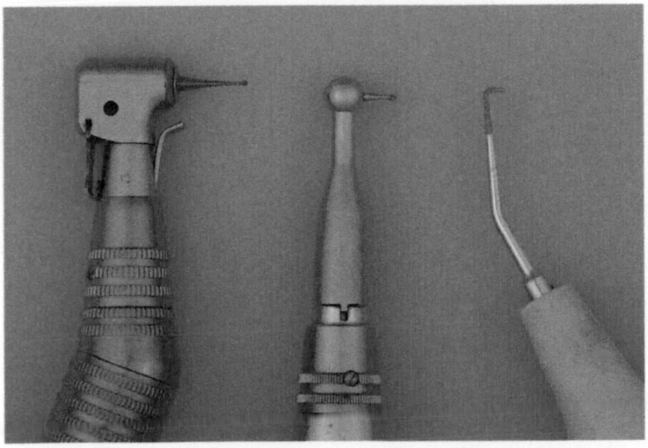

Figure 9.29 Size comparison (from left to right) of conventional contra-angle handpiece, microhead handpiece, ultrasonic-driven retropreparation tip.

easily allowing preparation along the long axis of the root. This provides numerous advantages over traditional methods of preparation (Box 9.6). Ultrasonic technology allows multiple bends in these cutting tips

Box 9.6 Summary of advantages with ultrasonic instruments for root end preparation

- Improved vision
- Better tactile feedback
- Smaller cavity preparation and more tissue conservation
- Easier to maintain preparation in the long axis of the root
- More thorough debridement of debris

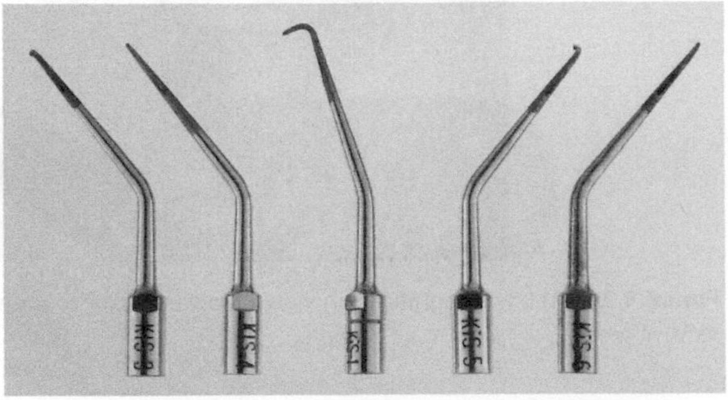

Figure 9.30 KiS microsurgical ultrasonic tips. Designed for different areas in the mouth, these tips have an irrigation porthole close to the cutting end for cooling.

(Fig. 9.30) to enable root end preparations to be carried out in all areas of the mouth and still maintain a preparation in the long axis of the root. In addition, narrow designs are available for running out isthmus areas which are now considered to be a previously unrecognized reason for failure in multi-canalled roots.

In many situations it is helpful to start off preparation using a sharp CX1 explorer, creating a tracking groove to provide a pathway for the ultrasonic tip. Alternatively, a series of small dots can be placed along an isthmus, using a light touch on the ultrasonic device, without water for improved visibility. These may then be joined together with the ultrasonic tip, using water spray for debridement and cooling. These actions help to ensure the retrograde cavity is prepared appropriately down the long axis of the canal. Care needs to be taken with the power settings during use; ideally, they should be used initially at low power, only increasing it as necessary. Such an approach will produce an ideal retrograde cavity with minimum risk of root cracking.[14]

Excess softened gutta-percha should be removed prior to vertical condensation with a microcondenser.

This should be repeated until a cavity depth of 3 mm is reached. This means that the apical 6 mm of the root is treated (Fig. 9.31). Subsequently, 3 mm of the root end in which it is thought that microorganisms are harbouring is removed, and a further 3 mm is cleaned and debrided to enable a filling material to seal the root end and prevent further reinfection of the periradicular space. Before placing any root filling, ensure that the base of the bony crypt is packed with Racellets or Telfa pads, so that any excess material can easily be retrieved, as previously explained.

Root end filling materials

Over the years there have been numerous different materials used for root end fillings. Amalgam was the first choice retrograde filling material for many years. However, it has become unpopular, due to the development of new materials, its mercury content, soft tissue staining and corrosion. Although a multitude of materials are used, all demonstrate signs of leakage, hence the importance of thorough canal debridement and obturation. Currently, the favoured retrograde material is mineral trioxide aggregate (MTA; Fig. 9.32). Other materials that have proven success are immediate restorative material (IRM) and Super EBA.

MTA is a material very similar to Portland cement and was developed in the 1990s by Torabinejad and colleagues. It has excellent sealing properties[15] and biocompatibility.[16] As it sets in a hydrophilic setting reaction, moisture control is not as critical as it would be for other materials; however, it can be difficult to handle. Super EBA is easier to handle and can be rolled into a small cone so it can be picked up on a flat plastic or a Hollenbach instrument and placed in the retrograde cavity; IRM can be handled in a similar fashion. MTA may be deposited in the root end cavity using a carrier such as the Dentsply MTA gun (Fig. 9.33) or one of the Dovgan MTA carriers (Fig. 9.34). One must take care not to place too much material in the barrel of either carrier as this may require excessive force to extrude the material and lead to its blockage or fracture. The material is lightly packed down following placement and then condensed using indirect ultrasound. MTA is not easy to pack, in view of its sandy consistency, especially if the mixture is wet. Moulding

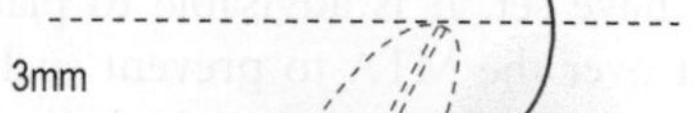

Figure 9.31 Root end resection, preparation and filling results in the apical 6 mm of root being treated.

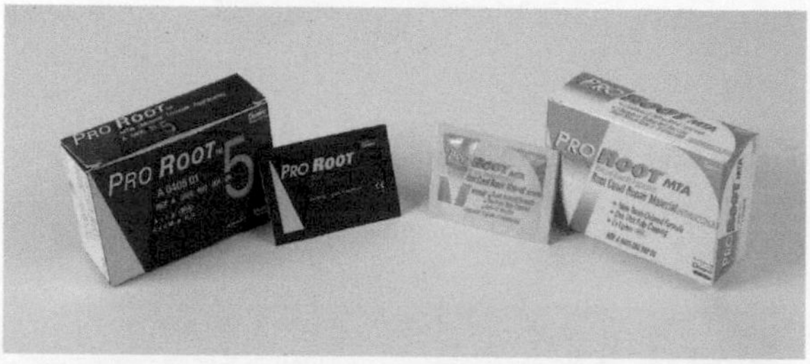

Figure 9.32 White and grey mineral trioxide aggregate.

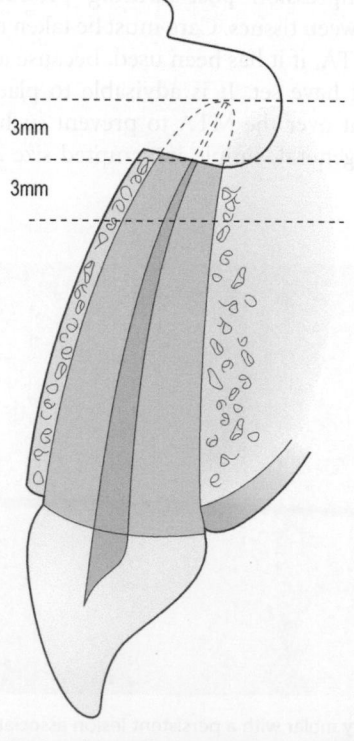

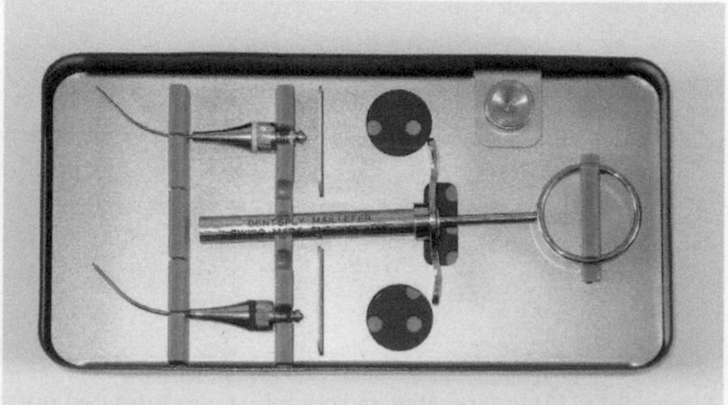

Figure 9.33 Dentsply MTA gun.

blocks are available to help form it into a cone so it can be used in a similar way to Super EBA. Work is also proceeding on an ultrasonic MTA carrier to simplify its placement.

It is usual to have some excess material overlying the root end following material placement. Super EBA or IRM can be trimmed back with a finishing bur once it has set. However, this is not appropriate for MTA, as its setting time is between 4 and 6 hours. Care must be taken to remove MTA from the root end around the retrograde filling. This may be performed with a small Ultradent brush used on the dentine surface and kept away from the filling to avoid saucering of the restoration. Ideally, a radiograph should be taken prior to suturing to ensure that the retrograde preparation and filling are adequate (Fig. 9.35).

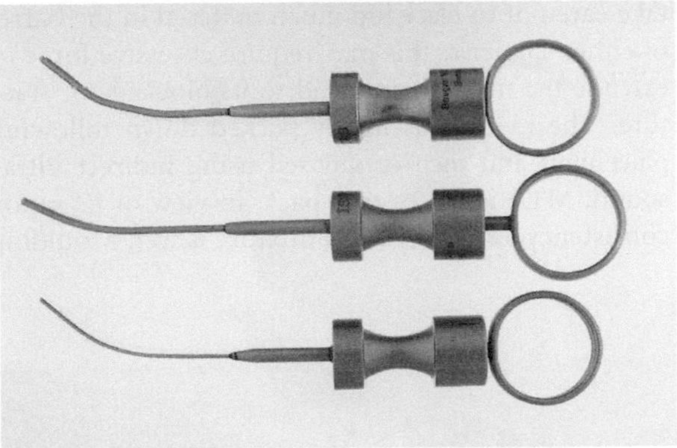

Figure 9.34 Dovgan MTA carriers.

When carrying out orthograde root filling, where it is considered highly likely that periradicular surgery may be indicated in the future, an 'apical plug' can be placed from an orthograde approach. MTA, Super EBA or IRM can be placed in the apical 6 mm and, when the root end is resected, 3 mm of previously placed material will remain. This material will have been placed under rubber dam and the canal irrigated with sodium hypochlorite just prior to material placement. This will mean that the remaining 3 mm of apical filling material will have been placed under more ideal conditions than from a retrograde approach. As a result, there will be no need for root end cavity preparation and placement of root end filling at the surgical phase.

Debridement and closure

The surgical area should be thoroughly debrided and the flap compressed for about 3 minutes prior to suturing and for a further 3 minutes after closure. Initial compression enhances intravascular clotting while compression post-suturing produces a thin hiatus between tissues. Care must be taken not to wash out the MTA, if it has been used, because at this stage it will not have set. It is advisable to place a plastic instrument over the MTA to prevent such an occurrence. In general, simple interrupted size 4/0 sutures

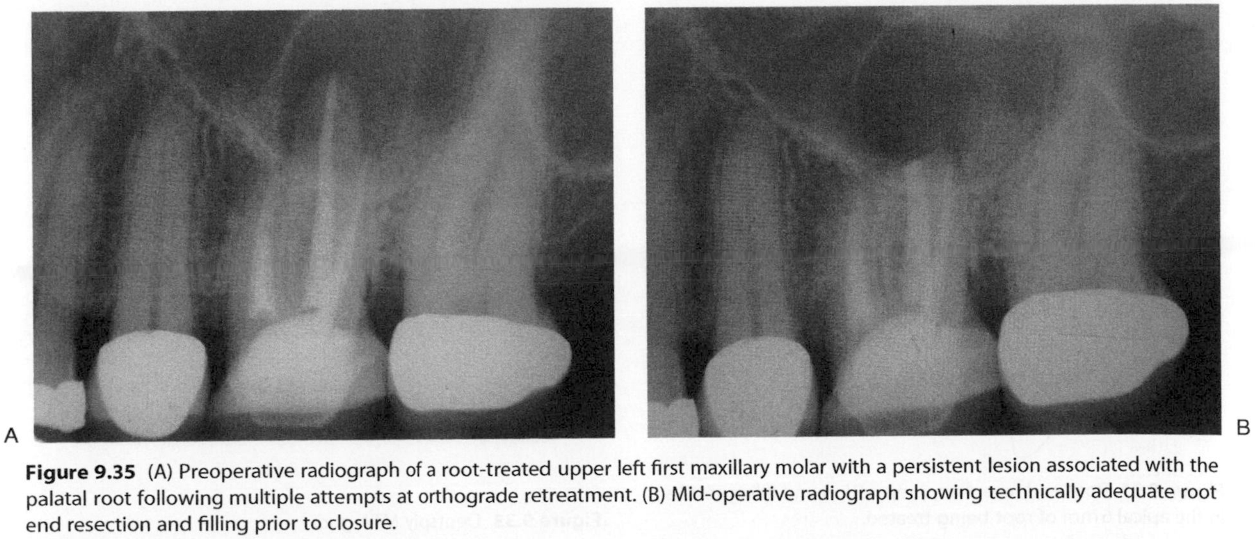

Figure 9.35 (A) Preoperative radiograph of a root-treated upper left first maxillary molar with a persistent lesion associated with the palatal root following multiple attempts at orthograde retreatment. (B) Mid-operative radiograph showing technically adequate root end resection and filling prior to closure.

will prove adequate for most situations, although some operators prefer to use 5/0 or even 7/0. Over recent years, suture material choice has moved from black silk to Tevdek braided polyester or monofilament polypropylene sutures such as Prolene.

Following periradicular surgery, consideration may be given for the use of guided bone regeneration (GBR) as an adjunctive therapy. GBR uses a barrier membrane to prevent undesired cells from invading a healing site and, and at the same time, to maintain space for desired cells to proliferate during early healing. Dietrich at al[17] have demonstrated promising results following periradicular surgery in teeth with apicomarginal bony defects and the use of GBR techniques. However, there is limited evidence as to efficacy at this stage.

POSTOPERATIVE MANAGEMENT

It is usual for a patient to have some discomfort and swelling postoperatively. This is usually minimal and can easily be controlled using analgesics such as non-steroidal anti-inflammatory drugs.[18] If the procedure has been lengthy and one expects more postoperative pain than normal, a long-acting local anaesthetic — such as bupivacaine (Marcain), which lasts for up to 8 hours — can be used. The area should be kept clean with a twice-daily chlorhexidine mouthwash until healing and suture removal allow improved tooth-brush access. Sufficient healing will have occurred after 48 hours[7] for suture removal; however, it should not be left longer than 96 hours due to the 'wicking' effect that may cause postoperative infection of the surgical site.

It is possible for ecchymosis to develop extraorally, and patients should be warned of this; however, it is self-limiting and will usually resolve in less than 2 weeks. If the site becomes infected and systemic signs such as pyrexia and regional lymphadenopathy are noted, then suitable antibiotics should be prescribed. All cases should be followed up at regular intervals, at least until healing is complete.

CORRECTIVE SURGERY

Corrective surgery may be required to seal a perforation or resect a root. The position of the perforation is of paramount importance in determining whether it is surgically accessible and parallax radiographs will help in determining this. Perforations in the apical third of the root may be handled by removal of the apex and sealing the canal with a retrograde filling. Ideally, perforations resulting from post crowns should have the offending post removed and a new one placed within the root canal. Surgical correction will then resemble the placement of a retrograde filling in the side of the root. If the post is not removed, then it must be cut back sufficiently to allow an adequate margin for finishing the retrograde filling. However, this is frequently problematic and a compromise may be necessary. Wherever possible, current practice prefers internal repair of root perforations.

Surgical root resection may be indicated on multi-rooted teeth that have not responded to treatment or have a hopeless periodontal prognosis. Other reasons for root resection include extensive resorption, root fracture or gross caries.

REFERENCES

1. Carr G B, Bentkover S K. Surgical endodontics. In: Cohen S, Burns RC (eds) Pathways of the Pulp, 7th edn. St Louis: Mosby, 1998: 616.
2. Rubinstein RA, Kim S. Long-term follow-up of cases considered healed one year after apical microsurgery. J Endod 2002; 28: 378–383.
3. Kim S, Pecora G, Rubinstein RA, Dorscher-Kim J. Colour Atlas of Microsurgery in Endodontics. Philadelphia: Saunders, 2001.
4. Danin J, Linder LE, Lundqvist G, Ohlsson L, Ramskold LO, Stromberg T. Outcomes of periradicular surgery in cases with apical pathosis and untreated canals. Oral Surg Oral Med Oral Pathol Oral Radiol Endod 1999; 87: 227–232.
5. Buckley JA, Ciancio SG, McMullen JA. Efficacy of epinephrine concentration in local anaesthesia during periodontal surgery. J Periodontol 1984; 55: 653–657.
6. Cutright DE, Hunsuck EE. Microcirculation of the perioral regions in the Macaca rhesus. I. Oral Surg Oral Med Oral Pathol 1970; 29: 776–785.
7. Harrison JW, Jurosky KA. Wound healing in the tissues of the periodontium following periradicular surgery. I. The incisional wound. J Endod 1991; 17: 425–435.
8. Velvart P. Papilla base incision: a new approach to recession-free healing of the interdental papilla after endodontic surgery. Int Endod J 2002; 35: 453–460.
9. Bender I B, Seltzer S. Roentgenographic and direct observation of experimental lesions in bone. J Am Dent Assoc 1961; 62: 152–160.
10. Lin LM, Gaengler P, Langeland K. Periradicular curettage. Int Endod J 1996; 29: 220–227.
11. Kim S, Endodontic microsurgery. In: Cohen S, Burns RC (eds) Pathways of the Pulp, 8th edn. St Louis: Mosby, 2002.

12. Vertucci FJ. Root canal anatomy of the human permanent teeth. Oral Surg Oral Med Oral Pathol 1984; 58: 589–599.
13. Gilheany PA, Figdor D, Tyas MJ. Apical dentin permeability and microleakage associated with root end resection and retrograde filling. J Endod 1994; 20: 22–26.
14. Waplington M, Lumley PJ, Walmsley AD. Incidence of root face alteration after ultrasonic retrograde cavity preparation. Oral Surg Oral Med Oral Pathol Oral Radiol Endod 1997; 83: 387–392.
15. Torabinejad M, Watson TF, Pitt Ford TR. Sealing ability of a mineral trioxide aggregate when used as a root end filling material. J Endod 1993; 19: 591–595.
16. Economides N, Pantelidou O, Kokkas A, Tziafas D. Short-term periradicular tissue response to mineral trioxide aggregate (MTA) as root-end filling material. Int Endod J 2003; 36: 44–48.
17. Dietrich T, Zunker P, Dietrich D, Bernimoulin JP. Periapical and periodontal healing after osseous grafting and guided tissue regeneration treatment of apicomarginal defects in periradicular surgery: results after 12 months. Oral Surg Oral Med Oral Pathol Oral Radiol Endod 2003; 95: 474–482.
18. Mehlisch DR, Sollecito WA, Helfrick JF et al. Multicenter clinical trial of ibuprofen and acetaminophen in the treatment of postoperative dental pain. J Am Dent Assoc 121: 257–263.

Index

Note: Page references in *italics* refer to Figures; those in **bold** refer to Tables or, if followed by the suffix **b**, to Boxes.

Printed and bound by CPI Group (UK) Ltd, Croydon, CR0 4YY

03/10/2024

01040365-0003